Call
the
Vet

BRUCE FOGLE

Call the Vet

My life as a young vet in 1970s London

HarperCollins*Publishers*

HarperCollins*Publishers*
1 London Bridge Street
London SE1 9GF

www.harpercollins.co.uk

First published by HarperCollins*Publishers* 2020

1 3 5 7 9 10 8 6 4 2

© Bruce Fogle 2020

Bruce Fogle asserts the moral right to be
identified as the author of this work

A catalogue record of this book is
available from the British Library

HB ISBN 978-0-00-842430-5
PB ISBN 978-0-00-842431-2

Printed and bound in Great Britain by
CPI Group (UK) Ltd, Croydon

To the kind staff and volunteers at Hearing Dogs for Deaf People (www.hearingdogs.org.uk) who provide such incredible dog buddies for people, young and old, that find themselves isolated by impaired hearing. And to the diligent, dedicated people at Humane Society International, especially those in Canada (www.friendsofhsi.ca). You operate under the radar, sometimes in dreadful circumstances, but you do brilliant work defending animals worldwide.

INTRODUCTION

Another overcast, moody, gunmetal grey day. London, 1970. Drizzle. I am a 26-year-old Canadian, fresh out of the Ontario Veterinary College, working as an assistant in a veterinary practice in Knightsbridge in the heart of the city. I'm here because … well, I don't actually know why I'm here.

It's far from home. That's exciting. I speak their language, so I can make my way around, get a job, have fun. I think of myself as British. At home in Toronto I grew up singing 'God Save the Queen' as often as 'O Canada'. The Queen is on my Canadian money. I vote for Members of Parliament, not Congressmen. But three months in London has me questioning that assumption. What I'm learning is that although I share their language, I don't share how they think.

A distinguished looking man in his sixties, in a tailored pinstripe suit, brings in his dog, a sad, grey-faced, female black Labrador, for me to put down. Not a twitch of emotion from him. His mother comes with him. Except it isn't his mother. It's his nanny. Not his children's nanny. *His* nanny. The woman who looked after him when he was a child. Where is his wife? His grown children? Why is there no feeling, no passion?

I am already feeling a bit antsy today, a bit out of place.

'Bruce, I've received a complaint about you,' my boss Brian Singleton politely but firmly tells me when he arrives at his surgery. 'Meet me in my office at 8.45.'

I can't finish my coffee, can't do anything but go over in my mind all the dogs and cats I have seen in the last few days, trying to work out where I'd made such a grievous diagnosis that the animal's owner had gone out of their way to complain about me. I have limited clinical experience, so my confidence in my ability to diagnose and treat effectively is years away. At that time in my life, I still reacted to events. I didn't yet have the ability, the maturity, to understand that life is more likely to go in the direction you want it to go in if you make things happen, not just respond to stuff.

That's it, I think. *I've killed someone's pet, but if I go back to Canada now, I can start afresh and no one there will ever know what's happened.*

I meet Brian in his office.

'Bruce, the lady who you saw yesterday, Mrs Pilkington, has complained about your attire.'

'My clothes?' I burst with relief.

Brian wears a dark suit and tie to work and expects me to as well. I do. I have no problem with that. The Beatles wear ties. My own father wears a tie when he crawls under our summer cottage each spring to turn the water supply back on.

'She didn't like my tie?' I mock, and Brian replies, 'You were wearing sandals. She doesn't feel, nor do I, that sandals are appropriate footwear at a veterinary surgery.'

This is 1970. In Canada, I had flower decals on my car. My suits are velvet. My trousers have flares. My thick chestnut-coloured hair tumbles down my neck. Of course I wear sandals. How on earth could that be so reprehensible that someone would complain to my boss? And why would Brian agree?

I don't get it. It is another seed in my mind that although we speak the same language, there really is a gulf between the English and me.

I come from a demonstrative family. The Fogles can be reserved but my personality comes from my mother's side, the Breslins, and they don't do reserve. They can be loud. They laugh outrageously. They question authority. They argue for the simple joy of words. They cry liberally. And when you need emotional support, they're with you, like an infantry platoon of aunts, uncles and cousins.

So when it comes to putting down this Labrador, the dog's sweet, gentle face looking up at me, at her owner and at her owner's nanny, I feel just awful. Why doesn't the owner feel as upset as I do? How can this man be so cold on such a poignant day, when his dog is to die? Why isn't his family with him? *What is it with you Brits?*

I was in my twenties before Canada had her own red maple leaf flag. The schools my brother and I went to in Toronto, Allenby Public School and Earl Haig Collegiate, both named after World War I British field marshals, flew either the Union Flag or the Red Ensign, a flag with the Union Flag in the corner and Canada's coat of arms on its red background. English-speaking Canadians of my era were raised more British than the British. The Queen was my queen. Britain's Parliament was the mother of all parliaments. I read Rudyard Kipling and Thomas Hardy at school. I knew the names of every British prime minister of the twentieth century. That's why when I arrived in Britain, I thought I understood the British.

But inside I really wasn't British and part of me already knew that. My father was born in Glasgow, so I proudly claimed patriality (and I continue to feel a strong affiliation with Scotland). His family emigrated to Canada in 1907 when he was a year old, but enough of Scotland remained in him for him to

name me Bruce, my brother Robert and our dog Angus. My
father's grandfather, a blacksmith, was born in a town with
different names in German (Lasdein), Russian (Lozdzee), Polish
(Lozdzeije), Lithuanian (Lazdijai) and Yiddish (Lazdei). The
Fogles called the town Lazdei because they were part of the
great Jewish emigration out of Eastern Europe that began in the
1870s. My mother's family, the Breslins, were also part of that
biblical exodus. They came to Canada from what they called in
Yiddish Tolotshin, the Lithuanians called Talacynas, the Russians
Tolochin. They too were part of the Great Other that arrived in
Britain, the United States and Canada at the end of the nine-
teenth century. And as much as my parents' families had become
part of the weft of twentieth-century Canadian life, prominent
in medicine and business, I knew I was an outsider, that I wasn't
part of Canada's founding British or French heritage.

Seeing this man and his nanny, both seemingly emotionless,
the nanny telling the man to go out in the hall while I give his
dog a lethal injection, the man doing so without question, hits
me like a bolt. I'm not part of them. I don't want to be part of
them.

Yet I think I also intuitively understood even then that what
I was watching was a performance. An act. A veneer. Learned
behaviour. British theatre. I didn't yet fully understand how
deep the relationship can be between us and other animals, but
I instinctively knew it was impossible for this man not to feel
some emotion at the end of his dog's life, or for this woman not
to feel deeply for a man she had known since his infancy. There
is a common thread of compassion running through all cultures.
It is part of all of us.

It would also be years before I understood that the people I
was meeting in Knightsbridge were but a sliver of Britain's then
class-addled culture, a strand that, but for a few diehards (blow-
hards?), has now almost disappeared.

During the following decades, like some of Britain's colonial administrators, inch by inch I went native. (I see the same happening today with many of my American clients, posted to London by their financial institutions, initially despairing that Britain isn't America, then never wanting to leave.) It didn't take long, certainly no more than a decade, for me to accept the weather. Accepting the Brits, going whole hog and becoming British, took longer. It was easiest with, I hate to use the term, 'real people'. Almost the first Londoner to invite me out for a drink was Mick, one of the local dustmen. He was someone I could relax with. With other clients I saw at the clinic, it took longer for me to warm to them.

In my first years as a practising vet, I would discover that although I had a good grounding in the mechanics of medicine and how to sensibly diagnose and treat animals, I had no training at all in how to understand either my patients or the people who brought them to me. I didn't yet realise how uplifting pets are, how they make us smile and feel good. This is a story of how someone who was trained that animals have no feelings or emotions, at one of the best veterinary schools in the world, came to understand how dreadfully wrong that part of my education was. This is a memoir of my first years as a vet in what was the most exciting time and place to be one, London in the early 1970s. It is an outsider's view of the Britain that then existed, how that outsider went native and found a perfect home, and how caring for animals evolved from 'make do and mend' to the more sophisticated but not necessarily wholly better level it has reached today.

1

There is a rhythm to life that is greater than years. A natural order. We repeat our mistakes because evolution is too foolish to retain accumulated wisdom. But joyously we experience pleasures through ever-repeated personal discoveries: a dog's head on your lap, a cat rubbing against your leg. Life is exciting when we are young because there is so much to find out about. Some of us are lucky enough to continue to feel that way even when we are no longer young.

At the end of my formal education I was in London, embarking on, although I didn't understand it at the time, a transition in life. I could be doing what I 'should' be doing, what my family expected me to do, setting up life as a working vet in Toronto. But I wasn't. I still don't know whether I took the opportunity to come to London because it was an exciting prospect or because it was an opportunity to get away from my family, to be myself, whoever that was. A niggle in me says it was probably the latter.

Through a sequence of chances – a Canadian travel fellowship to work at Regent's Park Zoo followed by an unplanned meeting with Brian Singleton, a vet with a practice in central London – I was now on a two-year contract working for Brian. His surgery, five minutes' walk from Harrods, was from my

Canadian perspective a tired, old shoebox, although I soon learned it was better equipped than most other London surgeries. On the corner of Pont Street and Cadogan Lane, the only indication that it was a veterinary surgery was a seven-by-nine-inch brass plaque with the words 'Woodrow & Singleton Veterinary Surgeons' on it. That was the maximum size allowed by the Royal College of Veterinary Surgeons (RCVS), and as Brian was president of that organisation, he knew and respected the regulations. The RCVS was, in effect, the vet's union. Only union members could practise veterinary medicine and I had become a member, an MRCVS. That was a wonderfully grand way to add five letters after my name by doing no more than pay my union fees.

The reception room's two frontages of ceiling-to-floor shop windows were defended by always closed yellowing Venetian blinds. Marbled blue linoleum covered the floor. Four fluorescent strip lights clung to the ceiling. It never smelled of animals, only of cigarette smoke wafting from the bookkeeper's office to the right of the reception area. Along each windowed wall were four grey plastic and metal chairs. By the back wall was the receptionist's desk, with a passageway immediately to its right to the narrow stairs leading to the first floor 'consultation' rooms. I thought it endearing that we 'consulted' rather than 'examined'. To the right of that passageway were even narrower stairs leading to the basement housing the kennels, treatment and operating rooms. X-ray developing was in a cupboard on a landing going downstairs. The X-ray machine itself was in the bookkeeper's office. When I wanted to take an X-ray, she vacated and puffed in reception.

There is something inherently good about people who choose to spend their discretionary income caring for pets. That too was a discovery that would take time to make. You can rightfully argue that pets parasitise our hardwired, lifelong need to nurture. But if that's your argument, then house-plants and gardens are parasites too. For whatever reason people kept pets, from my first experience in clinical practice I enjoyed meeting owners as much as I did their pets. That doesn't mean I understood them or found everyone easy to deal with.

Appointments were scheduled at fifteen-minute intervals, with the nurse on reception buzzing me upstairs via the inter-com phone with who was next. Pat House, Mr Singleton's head nurse, buzzed me. Mrs Wax has arrived.

'Oy vey, those stairs,' Mrs Wax exclaims as she walks wearily into my consulting room, carrying her dogs' medical files, given to her by Pat.

'I'm only seeing you because Mr Singleton isn't here,' she says, handing me the files.

It's true that some people look like their dogs. Dogs are extensions of our personalities, although occasionally they also fill gaps – they behave or look the way we would like to if we could. Mrs Wax is a woman with a shiny helmet of lacquered black hair, not one strand of which I bet is ever out of place. Her three black toy Poodles follow at her heels, keeping her between them and me. They have their hair cut for showing and look like canine topiary. Back then, I thought that a dog's hair coiffed into pom poms and rosettes was no more than just stupid looking. It didn't take much time before I realised those haircuts were demeaning to what is a dazzling breed of dog.

Another thing. Mrs Wax is Jewish. I *know* her, where she is from, how she behaves. I might not understand other people I meet but I understand her. Her home looks like Versailles, except all the furniture is covered in plastic. If she has a daugh-ter, my parents will steer me elsewhere. With their ancestry in the Baltic States, my parents' families pretentiously look down on '*Fiddler on the Roof*' Jews, the ones with a passion for gold-plated water taps. They are 'nouveau'. That was a way of thinking I hadn't yet completely lost.

'Mitzi has kennel cough,' Mrs Wax tells me.

'How do you know?' I ask, trying to mask the superiority I feel. I am the professional she has come to for advice. She is simply Mitzi's owner and I think she shouldn't make her own diagnosis.

'How do I know? Do you need a veterinary diploma to know when a dog has kennel cough? I showed her last week. There was a coughing dog. She's coughing!'

'Putz!' I hear her mutter under her breath.

'Are they all coughing?' I ask.

'No, young man, but they will be unless you do something.'

'Let's have a look and a listen,' I say, and ask Mrs Wax to lift Mitzi onto the examination table. As she does so, Mitzi produces a soft, moist cough.

I look at Mitzi's file and see she is eight years old and spayed. Her two younger canine companions, also females, are not spayed.

Mitzi's eyes are bright, her teeth surprisingly clear of tartar and her ears devoid of the forest of hair I expect to see. The glands in her neck feel normal, but when I pinch her windpipe she gags and coughs, a cardinal sign of irritation typically caused by one of the bacteria or viruses that, lumped together, get called 'kennel cough'.

I put my stethoscope in my ears and listen to her lungs. They sound moist and fruity. Then I concentrate on her heart, and the valve sounds are muffled and loud. I have a 33 rpm LP of canine heart sounds that I'd brought with me from Canada. This is my cutting-edge continuing education and according to that LP, Mitzi has a grade six out of six heart murmur. The maximum. She is in the earliest stage of heart failure.

'Let's have a listen to the others,' I say, and when I examine them, their hearts and lungs sound normal and they just look at me querulously as I pinch their throats.

'Mitzi may have picked up kennel cough at the show and the others might be incubating it, so tetracycline antibiotics and honey in their water can help. You should keep them away from other dogs for the next three weeks. No dog shows. But Mitzi has a loud heart murmur. She's coughing because she has heart disease and her heart's not coping very well.'

Mrs Wax looks shocked.

'That's impossible. She just won the Veteran Class. Last week! The judge said she is in excellent condition. Where's Mr Singleton? I want to see Mr Singleton.'

'He's working at the Royal College today, but he's back tomorrow. I'd like to start Mitzi on digitalis and Lasix* now and you can see Mr Singleton tomorrow.'

'Don't you start any treatment until I know what's wrong with my dog!' she warns. 'I want a real vet, not some apprentice who doesn't know the difference between kennel cough and a heart attack.' She lifts Mitzi from the floor and holds her tightly to her chest. I am about to tell her it is important we start treatment today, but when I look at Mrs Wax's face, wet mascara is streaming from her eyes.

'I'll buzz Pat and arrange an appointment with Mr Singleton for tomorrow morning.'

When Brian offered me a job I asked my professor of surgery from Ontario, Jim Archibald, for his advice. Jim was on a year's sabbatical at the Royal College of Surgeons. 'Woodrow and Singleton is the best practice I know of,' Jim explained. 'It's a

---

* Digitalis is a heart medicine (found naturally in foxgloves) and Lasix was the brand name of the diuretic ('peeing' pill) furosemide. At that time, there was no generic alternative to Lasix.

good place to make your mistakes, four thousand miles from home.' He added, 'You'll establish a good ethical basis for your future.' Of course, I was too green to appreciate that Brian would have asked Jim about me.

Affable, angular Cuthbert Erskine 'Woody' Woodrow, then in his late sixties, godson of Lady Cadogan, was first president of the British Small Animal Veterinary Association, a relatively new organisation of companion animal vets that was less than fifteen years old. Its American equivalent, the American Animal Hospital Association, had been founded far earlier, in the 1930s. Woody had great presence but was also relaxed and approachable. He had just retired but still came in occasionally to do Saturday morning consults. Handsome, reserved Brian Singleton, in his late forties, was its third president, a world-respected orthopaedic surgeon and my boss. Vets in Canada wore white lab coats or green scrub tops when they examined pets. Woody and Brian consulted in dark Savile Row suits.

The following day, Mrs Wax returns and sees Brian, who admits Mitzi for more tests. After I finish my morning consultations, I go downstairs, where Mitzi is housed in one of the recently installed stainless steel kennels, not in isolation.

'Bruce, the patient doesn't have Battersea Cough.'*

Brian never calls pets by their names. They are always 'patients'.

'I've given her 20 milligrams of Lasix,' he says. 'Pat, please walk her in the mews every hour. Bruce, take lateral and VD

---

* Dogs taken to Battersea always picked up a cough while there but it wasn't caused by the known cause of 'Kennel Cough', a bacterium called *Bordetella bronchiseptica* (a relative of *Bordetella pertussis*, which causes whooping cough in us). Twenty-five year later it was discovered that 'Battersea Cough' is caused by a canine respiratory coronavirus. Although a vaccine was developed it was never licensed for use in dogs.

X-rays of the chest.' VD means 'ventrodorsal', with Mitzi on her back. He then goes back upstairs to attend to Royal College matters.

'Did Mrs Wax give you a hard time yesterday?' Pat asks as I carry Mitzi up from the basement to the X-ray room.

'She didn't believe my diagnosis,' I answer.

'That's because you look like you're fourteen,' Pat giggles.

In 1970, the Royal College of Nursing refused to allow the word 'nurse' to be used by anyone other than a member of that association, so ever-smiling, over-permed Pat was a Registered Animal Nursing Auxiliary, or RANA, one of the first, the even-keeled mother-hen of Pont Street. Assisting Pat was Jane, a younger RANA, and Brenda, a trainee.

'You'll look old soon enough after dealing with the people you'll meet here,' she smiles, as we enter the accountant's smoke-filled room to use the ex-hospital X-ray machine.

'Gertrude, we'll just be five minutes,' Pat tells the surgery accountant, who picks up her pack of cigarettes and lighter and leaves to have another cigarette in the waiting room. Gertrude, in her late fifties with skin like cracked china, is also the receptionist when the RANAs are busy with pets. She reminds me of the Wicked Witch of the West in *The Wizard of Oz*. Throughout my time at Pont Street, I simply avoid her.

We don lead aprons and while Pat holds Mitzi, I place the X-ray cassette on the table then pull on lead-lined gauntlets and take Mitzi back while Pat adjusts the machine's settings. I lay Mitzi on her side, stretching her out, and when the dog stops coughing, Pat, standing behind me, clicks the dial in her hand. I place a new cassette on the table, stretching Mitzi out once more, this time on her back, and once more when her coughing stops, Pat clicks.

Speaking soothingly to Mitzi, telling her what a good girl she is, Pat takes her back to her kennel while I stop off at the darkroom, the closet on the stairs landing, and under a red light remove the X-ray film from the cassette, slide it in a hanger, then dip it in developer until it looks developed, then in water and finally fixer. I hang the X-rays over a radiator until they are dry and go back downstairs.

'So how do I make myself look older?' I ask Pat.

She smiles back and after a pause replies.

'Have an unhappy love affair.'

'No. Be serious. What should I do to make people see that I know my medicine?'

Pat pauses once more, then looks up at me and with a seriousness I haven't seen before replies, 'You vets are taught that dogs and cats are cases. Well, they're not. They are family. People's sons and daughters. Their husbands and wives. Don't preach to people. Listen. Then they'll think you're older.'

That isn't the first important lesson I learn from nurses. Long before vets understood what was happening in small animal clinics, nurses knew. My profession is still, by culture, masculine.

The X-rays show typical changes brought on by valvular heart disease, fluid throughout the lungs. After Brian looks at the X-rays, he asks me to join him when he meets with Mrs Wax and a discharged Mitzi.

Pat brings Mitzi to his room. 'Mrs Wax, as soon as you left I immediately gave the patient an injection of Lasix to clean her lungs,' says Brian. 'It would have been much better if this had been done yesterday as my colleague suggested. I asked Dr Fogle to examine her lungs this afternoon, and he tells me the injection is already working and her heart cough will continue to improve this evening.'

Brian moves to the X-ray viewer mounted on the wall, where both X-rays are backlit.

'Mrs Wax, Dr Fogle was able to diagnose the patient's heart disease without the need for X-rays. You will see how large her heart is,' and he points out the bulge in the shadow on the left side. 'You will also see that the patient's lungs, that should be dark indicating air, are white indicating congestion. Dr Fogle was able to determine this yesterday by listening to your dog's breathing sounds.'

Mrs Wax has taken Mitzi from Pat and is holding her tightly. I say nothing.

'What about her kennel cough?' she asks Brian.

'Complete the course of tetracycline that Dr Fogle advised. If we're lucky, the other dogs won't need any treatment. Pat will give you this, and the medicines for her heart. I would like to see her again in a week. Dr Fogle has experience interpreting ECGs and has recommended that we acquire a machine. He will run an ECG on Mitzi when we see her.'

After she leaves, I turn to Brian. 'Thanks for that. Are we really getting an ECG?'

'We are now. Mrs Wax may be tricky but she's influential in the Kennel Club, and it's best to keep her in the tent. And Bruce, I don't know how to interpret ECGs, but you're a fresh graduate so I expect you do. And if you don't, I want you to know how to by next week.'

I waltz out of his room. I think Brian is scary but know that even though I'm in London, away from my family, at least professionally, I've got my own infantry platoon behind me.

2

There is a lyrical fantasy that vets are more clever than doctors because our patients can't tell us what's wrong with them. That may not be true, but you'll have a hard time finding a vet who will argue against it. Another trope is how we actually use the verbs 'to vet' and 'to doctor'. 'To vet' is to make a careful and critical examination of something, while 'to doctor' is to change something in order to trick somebody, or to add something harmful. What would you like to be known for? As a Canadian vet in London, I was able to have the best of both worlds. While UK vets graduated with bachelor's degrees and so were *Mr, Ms, Miss or Mrs*, Canadian vets graduated with doctorates so I could rightly claim to be a *Dr*. And I did, certainly for a year or so until I realised it created a barrier and I was happier with people calling me Bruce.

A common feature of my extended Canadian family is that we don't swear. None of us: my parents, siblings, aunts, uncles or first cousins. My kids don't either. Swearing was a cop-out. As teenage smart alecs, we sometimes used French-Canadian swear words, *sacrement or tabarnak*, but that was really to show each other how clever we were. When I got frustrated by the antics of my closest cousin, I'd call him a *toton,* a complete idiot, but never a 'tit'. I spent the first 25 years of my life hearing an occasional 'darn' or 'holy moly' and not much more. Then I arrived in Britain.

Brian didn't like going on home visits so I went on all of them, several each week so early one afternoon on a leaden, monochrome day I am standing on the pavement in Berwick Street Market in Soho, on a home visit to see two Dobermans that have drawn blood from each other in a lunchtime dispute.

After morning appointments finished, I'd exchanged a luncheon voucher, given to me instead of cash as part of my weekly salary, for a Scotch egg from Express Dairy, and with my mock leather doctor's bag filled with what I thought I'd need, I'd walked past the regal Royal College of Veterinary Surgeons headquarters in one of the great mansions in Belgrave Square, up past the ambulance entrance at St George's Hospital at Hyde Park Corner, along Piccadilly to cacophonous Piccadilly Circus. I continued past the theatres on Shafetsbury Avenue until I reached the bustling street market. I love that walk. Still do.

'Woodrow and Singleton' had a cream-coloured Morris Minor estate or 'shooting brake', as Brian called it, that I could use on home visits, or I could take taxis if I wanted. But if I had the time, I walked. That's a habit I haven't lost. I looked at the grand buildings I was strolling past and it was exciting to think they were older than the country I was from. It was like walking through an old black and white movie – recognisable but still alien.

I haven't been to Berwick Street Market before. Awnings from the Georgian shops and houses that line the street overhang the tarpaulins that roof the individual fruit and veg stalls, each lit by one or two naked light bulbs. Dogs – all mutts – lie on the pavement or simply wander around. They probably belong to stallholders. I don't know and don't ask. The stallholders shout out the prices of their produce, although at the

Shaftesbury Avenue end of the market there is one stallholder selling used clothes and another old fur coats and stoles, neither of whom give away their prices. I walk along the pavement until I get to the address I've been given, a tailor's shop, and press the buzzer for Flat Two. I notice the sign beside the buzzer says, '*Cindy – Large Chest for Sale*'. I think to myself that if I had a large chest for sale, I'd make a big, proper sign, glue a Polaroid of the chest on it and have it on my front door at eye level, not little and faded beside the bell.

An elderly Italian woman answers the door.

'Hi, I'm Bruce Fogle, the veterinarian,' I say.

'Meester Veta. You comma with me,' she replies, and I follow her up the stairs. I know from visiting my dad's relatives in Glasgow that the British don't like bright light, but the naked red bulbs in the hallway and landing cast no light at all, and I hope Cindy doesn't have them in her flat too. I won't be able to see which parts of the Dobies are bleeding and which aren't.

She opens a doorway from the hall into a room overlooking the market. I don't see any chests of drawers in that room.

'You waita heera, Meester Veta,' the old woman commands, and of course I do. I've always done what I'm told to do, although with time I've learned to question authority.

Good, I think. *At least there's a little natural light through the net curtains.*

'Miss Sharona!' she calls out. 'Meester Veta issa heera.'

'Thank fuckin' god!' Sharon replies.

'Come in, darlin',' she calls out, and I walk through the door into a tiny, narrow kitchen where two female Dobermans are curled like black commas on blue linoleum floor identical to the flooring at Pont Street. Neither gets up to greet me. Both look sad, some would say embarrassed, as dogs are so capable of appearing.

'I knew when the butcher gave me them bones there'd be trouble. They was real miserable wiv each other, a real cat fight.'

'Hi. What's her name?' I ask, as I lean down by the dog nearest me.

'Joni,' her owner answers.

I say hello to Joni, and when she shows no resentment to my touching her head I feel around her neck for signs of damage. My fingers land on raw flesh on the far side. She'll need a stitch-up.

I move over to the other dog.

'And her name?'

'Jayni. You know what fuckin' sisters are like, luv. Was a real cat fight.'

Jayni is just as calm as her sister, and when I call out her name she gets up, walks over to me and presses her head against my legs, asking to be touched. She limps, and I see two clean, oval puncture wounds on her front leg near the elbow. She flinches when I touch the leg but shows no aggression towards me, only that mournful look. Dobies have an unfair image as aggressive dogs. That's wrong. Many are real mamma's babies. I open my leather doctor's bag, get out my stethoscope and listen to Jayni's heart, then Joni's. Both are fine.

'Sharon, I'm just going to give Jayni some antibiotics. Her wounds will heal. They're easy for her to lick, so they'll stay clean. Joni needs stitches. I can do that here if you like, but I'll need you to hold her firm for me.'

'A proper nurse, I am,' Sharon tells me and I open my bag, take out a glass cylinder of xylocaine and drop the local anaesthetic into its metal syringe gun, then add a needle.

'Fuckin' 'ell! She won't like that!' Sharon blurts out.

'It's a very thin needle. I'll drip local anaesthetic over the wound, then inject around the edges.' I do this, first cleaning the area using cotton wool wetted with disinfectant. Then I rinse the wound with surgical spirit. Joni flinches but shows no anger.

While I prep, instil and clean, the transistor radio beside the sink plays in the background. In 1970s London I'd expected radio stations to play mostly British songs but Radio Luxembourg, the station Sharon has tuned into and the one I listen to in the sparsely furnished flat above the surgery where I am living, plays mostly American music. Today, it is cringe-making stuff, Lee Marvin singing 'Wand'rin' Star', then Norman Greenbaum's 'Spirit in the Sky'.

'I'm glad she's a Dobie. I don't have to clip any hair. It's a clean, fresh wound.'

From another compartment in my bag I take a spool of black surgical silk, cut off the length I need and thread it on a long needle with a curved cutting tip. I know from the last time I used that needle that it is getting blunt and is due for replace-ment. I place a long, narrow stainless steel bowl on the floor, part fill it with surgical spirit and drop a pair of scissors, a needle holder and the needle and silk in it. Nowadays, all of these items come in pre-sterilised packets.

Joni is an angel. The local anaesthetic works and she stands stoically, with Sharon on the other side of her from me, one arm around her neck by her head to slow down any snap she might make if I accidentally hurt her, and one arm around her chest. I think of how I love dogs. They're so much more noble than we are.

'That's the singer what Joni is named for,' Sharon says as I sew. Paul Burnett the DJ is playing Joni Mitchell's 'Woodstock'.

'I actually heard her live a few summers ago, at a bar called Le Hibou in Ottawa, with Leonard Cohen,' I comment.

'You finished yet, darlin'?'

The wound is a hanging flap and stitching is simple, first a holding stitch at the apex, then filling in on both sides.

Doberman skin is supple, but with a blunt needle I have to push ever harder with each stitch to complete the job. After I finish, I give both dogs their injections of Pen-Strep antibiotics and fill an envelope with pain-reducing phenylbutazone tablets, bute,* that will last for two days.

'That's wonderful, luv. It starts to get busy here around five. Now I don't have to be away from work. How much is it?'

I answer two guineas for the home visit and five pounds for the stitch-up and injections.

'Fuckin' hell. You make more by the minute than I do!' she replies.

Sharon takes seven green one pound notes and two shillings from a jar in the kitchen cupboard and gives them to me. I thank her and we walk back into her front room where a man is sitting on the sofa reading the *Daily Mirror*.

He looks up, stares blankly at me, then a wide grin bursts across his face. 'Dr Fogle! Fancy meeting you here an' all.'

I have no idea who he is.

'Don't you remember me? I brought the dogs to you to get 'em Epivaxed when Sharon was busy an' all.'

I still don't recognise him. At that time in my career, I was so concerned about the worthiness of my diagnoses and treatments, all I ever saw were the animals, never the people who accompanied them.

'Oh, yes. Hi. How are you?' and I shake his hand.

'Miserable buggers!' he says nodding his head towards the dogs in the kitchen. ''Ad a dust-up, did they?'

'Yes, over a bone. They're okay but they gave each other a chew. Same breed. Same age. Same sex. They tick all the boxes for having fights with each other. Do you know them?'

---

* More efficient pain-reducing 'non steroid' anti-inflammatory drugs will not become available for another 20 years.

'They're mine. They live wiv Sharon when she's workin'. They're here for protection.'

What does she need protection from, I think, and only then work out why the lights in the hallway are red. I turn to Sharon. 'If either one of them goes off her food, phone the surgery. They'll need more antibiotics. The stitches can come out in 10 days. I can send a nurse to do that or you can bring Joni to the surgery.'

'Mick'll bring her in for her stitches,' Sharon answers. I shake Mick's hand and Sharon walks me to the door and out into the hallway where I shake hers.

I start down the stairs, then stop and turn back to Sharon.

'Sharon, one more thing.'

'Yes, luv?'

'Any chance you can show me that large chest of yours?'

I'm as pleased as punch that I can do irony too.

3

Sensible people get pets directly from breeders and see litters of puppies or kittens with their mothers. In 1970s London, upper-class families often got their dogs from friends, the middle class got their dogs and cats mostly from pet shops, while the working class got theirs from unplanned litters or from Club Row, a Sunday street market at the top end of Brick Lane in the East End. Two pet shops, Town & Country Dogs and Harrods' pet department, were vital customers for Brian. There were two distinct types of dogs in Britain, purebreds and mongrels. Although mutts or mongrels made up the vast majority of Britain's dogs, at Brian's clinic well over half of the dogs I met were purebreds. It was an era where 'well-bred' people provided homes only for 'well-bred' dogs.

'Our most important client is Harrods,' Brian explains in my first week working for him. 'You will visit their pet department at lunchtime each Monday, whenever new stock arrives and whenever they ask you to. All new stock gets Epivaxed, and most important, you complete a partial vaccination certificate with the date of the animal's next Epivax with us. Our other important client is Jane Grievson at Town & Country Dogs. Her son Christopher Grievson brings their stock here to be checked and Epivaxed.'

Harrods was a nearby upscale department store, synonymous with the British upper classes and to my eyes fustier than the people they served. It flaunted its royal warrants, to Queen Elizabeth the Queen Mother for china, to Queen Elizabeth herself for 'provisions' or what I called 'groceries', and to the Duke of Edinburgh for 'outfits'. I called outfits 'clothes'.

Brian had an appointment system at the surgery. Most vets didn't.

'Time is important to our clients,' he tells me. 'They are not used to sitting around waiting. And they don't suffer fools gladly.' I don't know what he means by that. The term is too English for me, but I take it as a warning not to waste their time. 'And we don't socialise with our clients,' he continues. 'That compromises our relationship with them. No drinks after work. No dinner in their homes.'

As always, morning consultations started at 9 am and ran through to noon. It was a blazingly sunny and unexpectedly hot and humid summer Monday and I packed my medical bag with what I thought I might need for my weekly Harrods visit: stethoscope, thermometer, surgical spirit, a sterilised glass syringe, twelve needles and twelve doses of the dog vaccine Epivax.* I walked along Pont Street, across Sloane Street, through red-brick Hans Crescent to Harrods.

The pink buff terracotta building itself was so grand. Imposing, bronze-framed display windows and seven floors of expensive shopping, although not so expensive that I hadn't already bought myself a suit at the new, fashionable Way In department on the fourth floor. The dollars I had brought with me from Canada, that I used to supplement my meagre salary,

---

* The vaccine came with a two-inch serrated saw, to abrade the necks of the vials to make them easy to snap open. I routinely cut my fingers when snapping vaccine vials so I also took finger plasters for myself.

went a long way back then. I entered by the back door, at the corner of Basil Street and Hans Road, where chauffeurs stood formally by their Rolls-Royces, and took two stairs up at a time to the second-floor pet department and the Manager's office.

The Manager, a bushy-browed, beige man in his forties in a Viyella shirt, green wool tie and tan warehouseman's coat, with a rural accent that I sometimes found difficult to understand, formally greets me with a 'Good morrow, Vet. Do you wish to do rounds?'

With me leading, we systematically walk the aisles of his department, stopping first at the enclosure of baby alligators, where I scan their pen for any that look skinny or have removed themselves from the general cluster.

'The water looks a bit murky,' I comment.

'We are late changing it, Vet. It will be done.'

On their adjoining aisle the parrots, cockatoos, cockatiels and macaws are incredibly noisy. I look in each cage, at the inhabitants, at their food and water trays and at the floors to check the consistency of their droppings. I check the tanks of tropical fish for the health of the inhabitants and signs of excess feeding by the weekend staff, a common problem that might lead to contamination in a tank, and then on to the most enjoyable part of the department, the mammals. There are three skunks, a puma, and kennels filled with pups and kits.

'Where did you get the skunks?' I ask.

'We find homes for surplus stock from zoos,' the Manager explains. 'Three years ago we sold an elephant to the King of Albania.'

'I didn't know Albania had a king,' I say.

'I thought it was a posh area at the bottom of Savile Row,' he replies with a chuckle. A bit of irony there. 'But it's a country, and King Zog or his son lives in Switzerland. I know it's Zog because it rhymes with snog.' He chuckles again.

The skunks looks like they are six to eight weeks old. I am somewhat familiar with them, not just from their odour on my family's Yorkies after the dogs had been sprayed while chasing them, but from one I had found falling over in a creek and had brought home to nurse back to health. 'It probably has rabies,' my father told me when he came home from work, and he phoned Animal Control and had the skunk removed from our backyard.

'Did the zoo vaccinate them?' I ask.

'I will check on that, Vet,' the Manager says.

'What are you feeding them?'

'PAL and vegetables, Vet.'

'Good. Don't give them cat food. It's too rich for their livers. And the puma?'

'It's also surplus. We get them frequently. They sell well. This one arrived with the skunks.'

'What does it eat?' I ask.

'Fresh beef from the Food Halls, Vet.'

'Make sure it's beef on the bone,' I add. 'She needs calcium. And give her a tablespoonful of cod liver oil each day.' I had learned at London Zoo that big cats can suffer from Vitamin A deficiency, and cod liver oil was a well-balanced supplement.

I get down on my haunches, and the puma comes over and rubs her head against the inside of her enclosure. I put my fingers through the cage and feel the silkiness of her hair. 'That's a cat I'd be proud to be seen in public with,' I say.

'We had a lion cub here last year. I sold him for 250 guineas. Mind you, I would have given him away.'

'Why's that?' I ask.

'Sly creature, Vet. He got out one night and I found him over there in Carpets the next day. He'd shredded the goatskins.'

The last part of rounds today is the kitten and puppy kennels. There are no additions since my visit the previous week.

'The Persians sell well, but I am finding it difficult to obtain kittens, Vet. The breeders now want to sell them directly.'

The cat kennels are sparse, with one remaining Persian, two Siamese and two blue Burmese.

'Two litters of Yorkshire terriers arrive today, Vet. I hope they are here before you leave.'

Of the six Old English Sheepdogs I had vaccinated the week before, only two remain. They look surprisingly lonesome without their siblings, and stand on their hind legs wagging and smiling as I visually check them over. Beside them are four Dachshund pups, curled tightly together, and in the next kennel two Pug pups.

'Vet, the Pugs are sniffling.'

I rinse my hands with disinfectant, lift out the first Pug and listen to its chest. The heart and lungs are fine, and I hear referred noises coming from the throat.

'Her nostrils are so tight she has to breathe through her mouth,' I tell him. 'It's causing irritation in the back of her throat, and that's leading to her snorts and sniffles.'

Her littermate also has small nostrils.

'Do breeders send you Polaroids before you buy pups?' I ask.

'No, Vet. I know what sells best and I put in orders, although breeders ring me up when they have surplus stock they can't shift. If they're the right breeds, I'll buy them.'

'Okay, then. That's it?'

'As I say, I'd like you to see the Yorkshire terrier pups before you leave. Would you like a cup of tea? The train is due in at Paddington at half past the hour so they should be here momentarily.'

'Yes, fine. Thank you,' I answer and we walk through the 'Staff Only' door into a corridor leading to his office.

'Where are the pups coming from?' I ask.

'Most livestock comes from Wales, Vet.'

The Manager boils water in a kettle warmed on an electric ring and as it heats he adds several teaspoons of Harrods English Breakfast tea to a white teapot. He swirls the tea in the pot then pours it through a strainer into two flower-decorated teacups, and as he does so one of his shop assistants, a lean woman in her early twenties, with a brown fringe hanging over an intelligent face, comes to his door and says, 'The puppies have arrived, Sir. They're in the corridor.'

'Vet is having tea,' he replies.

'Thanks,' I say, 'I'll come and have a look now.' I pick up my medical bag and walk down the corridor to a large wooden crate with rope handles. There is no door.

'How do you open it?' I ask.

'The top is nailed shut so they can't escape,' the Manager says. He is carrying a claw hammer and, with the claw end, pries off the top. There is silence from inside the crate.

I look in. One pup sits up and unhappily looks at me. Another, with its hair pasted to its face by its own profuse saliva, lies on its side, glassy eyed, panting and drooling. A third pup is twitching and salivating. The rest are lifeless.

I pick up the sitting pup, give it a cursory look and hand it to the Manager. 'Put it somewhere with water.'

Without looking at her I say to the shop assistant, 'Get two of those fabric dog beds from the floor.'

I pick up the salivating pup and with my stethoscope listen to its chest. The heart sounds good. I listen to the twitching pup's heart. It sounds the same. I lift a lifeless pup and listen to its chest. No breathing or heart sounds. Then the next pup. It has a heartbeat. So does the next. So do all the rest. Only one is dead. I guess this is probably a low blood sugar crisis.

The shop assistant returns with the round fabric dog beds. The Manager places the healthiest pup in one of them.

'Do you have any maple syrup or honey for your tea?' I ask the Manager.

'I don't. But they do in the Food Hall. Come with me.'

I turn to the shop assistant. 'As fast as you can, run to the surgery, ask them for a vial of 50 per cent glucose and get back here, to wherever honey is in the Food Halls.'

'The surgery is on Pont Street, the other side of the lights,' the Manager adds.

I pick up the bed full of unconscious or frothing pups and follow the Manager across his department. He quick marches.

'Faster!' I shout and he moves from a brisk walk into a run, down the flights of stairs to the ground floor, through Menswear and into the Food Halls, straight to a selection of honey.

I take a jar from the display, open it, give it to the manager and say, 'Dip your finger in it and smear it in the mouths of the conscious pups.'

I take another jar and do the same with the unconscious pups, applying honey under their tongues and inside their cheeks.

'Animals are not allowed in the Food Halls,' I hear over my shoulder.

'These are not animals!' the Manager barks back. 'They are Harrods inventory!' No one seems upset that I have taken honey from the shelf without purchasing it.

It amazes me how fast sugar gets absorbed from the mouth into the bloodstream. The pups are small. They have little or no sugar reserve. They had been enclosed in a wooden crate since sometime in the early morning somewhere in Wales for a long, hot train journey to London before another hot ride in a taxi to Knightsbridge. I am burning with anger at how these pups have been treated, but I don't say anything.

The shop assistant arrives with the injectable glucose vial. I break it open and fill the syringe I have brought along to give vaccinations with, add a sharp new needle, place my finger on an unconscious pup's throat to raise its jugular vein, insert the needle and inject one millilitre of the concentrated sugar. Within a minute, the pup is moving and within five minutes sitting up. I do the same with the remaining two pups that have not responded to honey under their tongues. Both come back from the dead.

'Get me a towel, please,' I ask the Manager's shop assistant, and she instantly produces a tea towel. I give the brightest pup a rub then place it on the floor, where it gives a little shake that is too much for it and it sits down. I repeat the rub downs with the other five pups, and when I am convinced that their low sugar crisis is at least temporarily over, I put them in the dog bed and return with the Manager and his assistant to the second floor, this time by the lift.

'Oh, aren't they cute,' the lift operator says as we get in.

We return to the Manager's office.

'I'm sorry, I don't even know your name,' I say to him.

'Grimwade,' he replies. 'And this is Miss Clark.'

'Annabelle,' she adds.

In the corridor, the bed in which we placed the unharmed pup is empty when we return.

'Miss Clark, find that puppy,' Grimwade tells his assistant, and as he does so the pup scampers out from under his desk with a piece of wrapping tissue in its mouth.

I speak to them. 'Annabelle, please give that one a little honey with its dog food. Mr Grimwade, I'm taking these pups back to the surgery for the rest of the day. I want to make sure they're over their crisis. They shouldn't be left alone tonight.'

'Mr Grimwade, if you can arrange for a taxi I can take all of them home with me tonight. I can stay up with them,' Annabelle adds.

'We shall see,' he says.

'That's a terrific suggestion, Annabelle. Thank you very much. That's what we'll do. Mr Grimwade, considering the amount of money Annabelle saved Harrods with her Olympic-standard run to Pont Street, I think you can afford to provide her with the taxi fare home and back. I'll discuss the events with Mr Singleton, then give you written advice on where Harrods should get its puppies and kittens, how they should get here and what to do when they arrive.'

'I look forward to that, Vet,' Grimwade replies.

I think about asking him out for a drink that evening. I already know what I want to change in his set-up, but remember that Brian has told me no socialising, so I don't.

Back at the surgery, late in the afternoon, Brian calls me into his office.

'Bruce, may I introduce you to Mrs Jane Grievson from Town & Country Dogs and her son Christopher.'

Each has two Shih Tzus in their arms, a breed I have never heard of, let alone seen.

'Good afternoon,' they reply in unison.

Mrs Grievson has immaculately permed, bottle-blonde hair, is petite and vivacious, younger than my mother, an English rose whom I am instantly frightened of. Christopher, my age but more heavy set and a little taller, a man with an artlessly happy face, tickles the pups in his hands as his mother speaks.

'I was just thanking Mr Singleton for sending me to Mr Startup in Worthing. I was considering buying a new toy Poodle as a potential stud, and wise Mr Startup asked me to bring the pup's grandmother for him to examine. He found eye disease in the grandmother that he says is hereditary and leads to blindness, so I did not purchase the pup.'

Brian turns to me. 'There are no eye specialists at the Royal Veterinary College, but Geoff Startup in Worthing is very knowledgeable about eyes and sees referred cases.'

'And I was also telling Mr Singleton that you will be seeing more of Christopher,' says Mrs Grievson. 'My husband Bob and I enjoy dabbling in property. We have an old mill in Italy we are about to fix up.'

'Yes, I'm afraid so,' Christopher adds. 'Mother has convinced me to join her permanently. Bruce, have you visited our shop?'

I tell him I haven't and agree to visit after I finish the afternoon appointments.

'What type of pups are they?' I ask before I return to my list of clients, and I am impressed that Christopher answers before his mother can.

'They are Shih Tzus. Very rare. Oriental. We get them from a breeder friend of my mother's in Trevor Square.'

'We sell oriental breeds but we don't sell breeds to Orientals. They treat their dogs abominably!' Mrs Grievson adds.

Early that evening I walked up luxurious Sloane Street then left onto Hans Crescent. Town & Country Dogs was the second shop on the left, although its address is 35B Sloane Street. I assumed that Mrs Grievson managed to secure a better address because other people found her just as scary as I did when I'd met her a few hours earlier. I felt more relaxed when Christopher told me she had gone for the day and suggested that after a quick look around we go to a local pub for a drink.

The shop was elegant and feminine, with pastel, floral wallpaper, dark wooden floors, hanging lace in the north-facing windows that were set up for litters of pups to be displayed in and a pendant light fitting of smoked glass. Christopher takes me downstairs to see the pups' holding kennels and their clipping, washing and grooming facilities, then we walk over to the Nag's Head on Kinnerton Street, a mews street five minutes away.

'Have you been here before? It seems a suitably named drinking hole for a veterinary surgeon,' Christopher chuckles as he steps aside to let me enter the tiny, dimly lit, packed pub. The Nag's Head is simply a tiny mews house, no more than 15 feet wide, on a narrow lane, surrounded by private homes. It's like walking into someone's small, dark-panelled living room, 15 feet of standing room in front of a bar with stairs going down to the left and stairs going up to the right. The walls are densely covered in framed cartoons and art. I instantly fall in love with the place and decide that this will be my 'local'. I have a Carling Black Label, and we take our drinks outside and find room to stand between two parked cars in front of the pub. I had already learned during the shop tour that Christopher has the ability to speak so loudly and so fluently there are virtually no pauses where I can ask any questions.

'How did your mother come to set up Town & Country Dogs?' I spot an opportunity and Christopher embarks upon a resumé of his mother's life. Earlier that day, I had pigeonholed him as his mother's gofer. Now I hear the pride in his voice as he tells me the back story of the pet shop.

'My mother is not your typical British dog breeder. Much too glamorous.'

I'm relaxed with Christopher, so I ask, 'What's a typical British dog breeder?' and Christopher says, 'A woman who reached marriageable age just after World War I, found there were no men left to marry and so has devoted herself to dogs. Do you know Betty Conn Ffyffe? Wonderful woman. Enormous. Ever so loud. Only wears tweeds. Monocle. Barks ferociously. If a dog is reluctant to perform she shouts, "Pull yourself together," wanks it until it's blue in the face and two months later Mother has another litter to sell.'

I sip my ale and let his riff roll on.

'Mother has been breeding Poodles and Yorkies for over twenty years. After the War, her family – she lived in Kent – had nothing. She knew dogs and started out making clothing for them. Very upwardly mobile, she was. Mother saw that no one was catering to the top end of the market. She managed to convince *Tatler* to give her an enormous picture spread. That made her, her shop and her dogs well known to society. That's why we are around the corner from Harrods. Mother breeds most of the dogs she sells. She has an enormous facility in Cornwall. Or she knows breeders personally. But Bruce, you know what has really made the business so successful? Hollywood loves her. Simply adores her. They love her energy, her theatricality. Cary Grant or Ethel Merman or Elizabeth Taylor come into the shop and they think they are in an Edwardian film set, which is exactly where they are. We still can't find enough good Old English Sheepdogs for the Americans.'

'Is that why Harrods always has Old English Sheepdogs?' I ask.

'They get theirs from breed-to-order hill farmers in Wales. Dreadful places. Riddled with parasites. The pups don't meet a soul until they're put on a train to London.'

'Why Old English Sheepdogs though?'

'Because of Doris Day and David Niven and their Old English,' Christopher replies. 'In *Please Don't Eat the Daisies*, the film. It might be ten years old now, but it started a craze in America for Old English.'

'Did your mother supply the dog for the film?' I ask.

'It wouldn't surprise me, but I've never asked,' Christopher answers. 'Mind you, if she did, they would have had to pay for it then and there. Mother has very firm rules. No one is given extended credit, not President de Gaulle, not Princess Grace of Monaco.'

'They buy dogs from you?' I am impressed and wonder whether I'll meet them at Brian's.

'Yes, and they were not allowed to leave her shop until they paid for them. In full. In cash.'

'I'm trying to convince Brian to accept payment with Barclaycard,' I say, and I pull out of my pocket my Chargex credit card issued by my Canadian bank. 'It's identical to this, right down to the colours. Brian says it's only for shopping in department stores, but vets in Canada get paid this way and the card holder is liable if someone else uses it.'

'Too technical for mother,' Christopher replies. 'Cash rules.'

4

I talk with Brian about the low blood sugar Yorkies at Harrods and he asks me to give him in point form a short list of recommendations. With help from Christopher, I list:

- Wormed pups from reliable sources
- Bred for physical health
- Checked by breeder's vet before dispatch
- Open kennels for travel, accompanied by a person
- No crowding
- Sugared water available during transit
- Seen by us when arrive at Harrods.

Brian approves the list with one alteration:

- Seen by us at Pont Street before arrival at Harrods.

He asks Pat to flesh out each point into a single sentence, make two carbon copies and bring them to him for his signature. 'It's best that this letter comes from me,' he explains.

I tell him how good Annabelle the shop assistant was, and he says, 'Keep an eye on her. I think Jane is pregnant, and if she is we'll have to look for a new junior RANA.'

In the 1970s, pregnancy often meant you lost your job.

In the following weeks, I continued to do around twenty to twenty-five consultations each day, mostly dogs but some cats, a few birds and the occasional monkey or snake. At that time, I was too preoccupied with whether or not I was making accurate diagnoses to notice much about the owners, but I was aware they were mostly women and regardless of age almost invariably tall and well dressed. When I became more familiar with Britain's social orders, I realised that Knightsbridge acted like a magnet for tall, thin women. I imagine it still does.

I'd also noticed that we saw a large number of elderly Poodles owned by over-made-up, fleshy women, mostly in their late forties or early fifties.

'Those dogs can thank the Street Offences Act for the good lives they lead,' Brian tells me when I ask why Poodles had once been so popular.

'How's that?' I ask.

'The Act made it an offence for streetwalkers to solicit for business in public places. So the girls equipped themselves with Poodles. The dog's colour indicates the service its owner provides. They're mostly Shepherd Market Poodles. That's part of our catchment area.'

'So would you call them working dogs?'

Brian grinned.

My relationship with Brian was very much employee and employer. My instinct was to joke about what Brian had told me, but I didn't think I should so I didn't. In fact, I never relaxed enough with Brian to joke or make small talk with him about anything much. To a fresh grad like me, Brian was intimidating, more like a father figure you always wanted to prove yourself to.

Brian did all the complicated surgery, leaving me with mostly cat spays, dog and cat castrations and wound repairs, although I also did emergency ops and fortunately for me we saw lots of

emergencies when Brian was out of the surgery. His responsibil-
ities as Junior Vice-President of the Royal College of Veterinary
Surgeons were extensive, so Pat and I met all the pharmaceut-
ical company trade reps. I was obliged to stay at the surgery
most nights and alternate weekends to take telephone calls and
see any emergencies. If I wanted to go out in the evening, I
arranged with the Post Office telephone operator to answer
calls to us and refer them to Keith Butt, a vet in Kensington.

A nurse joins me in the surgery on Saturday mornings, and it
is Pat rather than Jane or Brenda who is on duty when a
distraught women bursts in with her rag of a little dog cradled
in her arms.

'Oh god, she's been attacked by an Alsatian! Please! Help!'

I am sitting on the corner of the reception desk idly talking
to Pat and can see visible flesh in the Maltese's chest. I take my
stethoscope from my neck to listen to its heart but before I have
a chance to do so, Pat takes the dog from the woman.

'I'm just taking her downstairs.'

I follow her down.

'Turn on the oxygen,' she tells me as she opens the dog's
mouth, inserts an endotracheal tube into its windpipe and blows
into it. I watch candy floss pink lung tissue inflate and bulge out
of the torn chest.

Pat continues to blow into the tube until I have oxygen flowing through anaesthetic tubing and she can breathe for the little
thing by compressing an inflated anaesthetic bag.

'Now you can listen to its heart,' she tells me, and I do. It's
beating perfectly.

'Where is Mr Singleton when you need him,' she says, more
I think to herself than to me.

I feel stupid, reaching for a stethoscope rather than doing
something to save the dog's life. Pat, the instinctively good
nurse, doesn't comment on my foolishness. I examine the ragged

wound and see that one lobe of lung is punctured and damaged beyond repair, but the others on the injured left side are untouched. Two ribs are broken. It is the dog's own rib that damaged her lung, not the Alsatian's teeth. Pat continues to inflate the dog's lungs by compressing the oxygen bag, but now with oxygen in her circulation she regains consciousness and is trying to get up.

'Add ether,' I tell Pat, and she opens the valve on the anaesthetic machine to run the oxygen through liquid ether. She opens the valve on the nitrous oxide cylinder and adds that gas to the mix. That settles the dog into anaesthetic unconsciousness.

'Give her pethidine,' I tell Pat.* Pethidine will lighten her breathing.

I tell Pat to continue 'bagging' the dog – inflating its lungs for it – while I prepare a tray of surgical instruments, and as I do we hear the telephone ring in reception.

'Everything's fine down here,' Pat calls through the closed door. 'Can you please answer that and get the caller's telephone number?'

'This is what's called on the job training,' she says, as I carefully cut away the little Maltese's long white hair that has been sucked into its chest and prep the surgical site. If the dog is to survive, I have to remove two ribs and one lobe of lung, sew off the air passage and lung tissue so that there is no leakage of air whatsoever, then sew up the chest wall air-tight, coordinating the last stitches going in with Pat inflating the repaired lung back to its maximum.

'I've done this before,' I say.

'Never!' Pat replies. 'At the zoo?'

_____

* Pethidine is a narcotic painkiller. It's still used sometimes but was succeeded by methadone.

'No. We had surgical exercises at college. I've done one of just about everything.'

As I scrub up, the Maltese's owner puts her head around the door to the prep room.

'May I come in? Is she all right?'

'She has dreadful injuries, but Dr Fogle is familiar with the surgery she needs and he's just about to start. If you can answer the door and the telephone, I can stay with her. Right now she needs me to help her breathe. This is Bianca, isn't it?'

'Yes, it is,' the owner says.

'Mr Singleton spayed her last summer. She's a sweety.'

'And you're Felicity Templeton-Ellis?' Pat asks.

'What a good memory you have.'

'Well, I do read the papers.'

My interest and competence in surgery had been honed back in Canada by Jim Archibald, my professor of surgery, who co-authored the textbook *Experimental Surgery* and edited the first surgery text for small animal vets, *Canine Surgery*. He was the dominant personality at the Ontario Veterinary College, and the curriculum committee gave him extensive time for his students to perform 'surgical exercises'.

He chose his favourite students, and I was one of them, to work their final summer at the College as salaried employees performing experimental surgery – taking a dog's kidney from the abdomen and transplanting it into the neck, opening a sow's belly then her womb, then her unborn piglets, punching holes in their diaphragms then sewing everything back together so that human obstetricians could try to keep the piglets – born with the equivalent of torn diaphragms – alive long enough for full-time surgeons to arrive to save them. I never thought about the welfare of the animals I was experimenting on, only the challenge of operating successfully.

For surgical exercises, each group of four students was given a dog and a sheep to operate on in alternate weeks. We would open the dog's abdomen – a 'laparotomy' – then sew her up, let the incision repair, then two weeks later do another laparotomy but this time remove her spleen then sew her up, play with her for another two weeks, then open her up again, open and close her bladder, then sew her up once more. As long as the dog survived we kept operating on her, removing a section of her intestines, or a kidney or a lobe of lung. If you think that what I was doing was barbaric, all I can do is utterly agree. What makes be shiver as I write this is that the welfare of these poor, innocent dogs never even entered my mind, or as far as I'm aware, the minds of my classmates. Most of us were men – only three women were accepted each year. Most of us were off farms or ranches, and those of us who weren't, including me, didn't have the basic thoughtfulness to question what we were doing. We *wanted* our dogs to survive to the next operation, to prove to Professor Archibald we were proficient surgeons. Being given a replacement dog was a sign of failure. What does that say about human nature?

I'm not saying that veterinary students should not practise on live animals. I am in favour of surgical exercises where a dog that is going to be killed because no one wants it is anaesthetised and operated on, then immediately killed without regaining consciousness. Today, I wasn't 'learning on the job' when I was confronted with the difficult surgery that Bianca needed if she was to survive. I had learned to do a lobectomy and rib resection on a stray dog that no one had a continuing emotional investment in. But I still don't fully understand why throughout my training as a vet I never once considered the welfare of the defenceless animals that I did surgical exercises on. They must have been family pets. Had they got lost? Were there families somewhere wondering what had happened to their dogs? How did the dogs feel? What did the dogs feel? It's just horrific.

Bianca's surgery is uneventful. We don't paralyse her breathing with curare-like drugs,* something we did during surgical exercises, simply because we don't have these drugs at the surgery. That means Pat coordinating the compression of the anaesthetic bag in synchrony with Bianca trying to take a breath herself. The challenge comes when we turn off her ether. The narcotic effect of pethidine keeps her breathing light, but even when she groans and screams, the stitches hold and her lungs remain inflated. By now the air in the operating room is heavy with ether that has seeped from Bianca's torn lung.

'We really should use halothane,' I say to Pat. That's the new and much safer anaesthetic gas we used at college.

'Tell Mr Singleton,' she replies.

While Pat wraps Bianca's chest in gauze bandage, I go upstairs to reception.

'She's not out of the woods yet, but so far so good,' I say to her owner.

'Can she come home?'

'Not today. I'll keep her with me upstairs over the weekend. I'm on call anyways. Give me your number and I'll call to give you progress reports.'

Felicity Templeton-Ellis writes down her number and gives it to me then says, 'How can I thank you? She means more to me than anything.' And she embraces me in a whole body hug and holds me tight.

Is this what Brian calls 'socialising with clients'? I walk her to and through the front door and return downstairs. Pat has

---

* Curare (from a tree bark) was used on arrow tips by South American people to paralyse prey. It works by paralysing motor nerves. Synthetic drugs were developed to do the same.

placed Bianca in a cage and fed an oxygen line into it. 'I'll keep an eye on her and you can write up her notes, then I can write up her invoice,' Pat says.

'I'm impressed,' she adds. 'You may look like you're fourteen but that was a job well done under fire. And fast. You should tell Mr Singleton you want to do more sophisticated surgery. And you'd like, what did you call it, halothane?'

'Yes, halothane. By the way, who's the owner?'

'She's part of the Clermont Set. Her husband is a notorious gambler. The *Express* says she is one of the most beautiful women in England.'

'I noticed,' I add with a smile.

I don't tell Pat but I feel like a hero. I'm brilliant! I'm omnipotent! No one else could have done that. That dog would have died without me.

In 1970, that's how I felt each time I saved a life. Now, with time and failures behind me, when I carry out a similar procedure there is satisfaction but with a far more profound feeling of humility. What I've learned is that when there are successful outcomes like with Bianca, and I make others happy, it can only lead to personal happiness and contentment. Success isn't just good for your patients and their families, it's just as important for our own personal happiness.

I kept Bianca upstairs in my flat above the consulting rooms over the weekend, on a bed of bath towels. These days, I'd keep her on painkillers for a week, but over fifty years ago we didn't give pets much painkiller. We were taught that pain was a perception and only humans were capable of the abstract thought needed to perceive it. Bianca cried and moaned as I expected her to do after surgery. Background noise in the kennel room – it's what all dogs did, though cats didn't, and it took my profession much, much longer to accept that cats too feel intense pain. They just don't vocally express it.

Bianca cried out each time I picked her up and carried her outside to the mews to let her empty her bladder. She lapped a little water on the Saturday evening but refused food until late Sunday, when she ate some Express Dairy sausage.

Today I lie on the floor with her. 'Good girly,' I tell her, and stroke her head. She looks up at me sadly, but then a tiny sparkle comes back into her eyes. I telephone Felicity with the good news, she comes to the surgery, picks up Bianca, and I arrange a home visit for Wednesday lunchtime.

'You should have kept her here,' Brian sternly tells me on Monday morning when I recount her injuries and surgery. His policy was to do all significant surgery, even simple dog spays, at the veterinary hospital built in the outbuildings of his home in Surrey. Every Tuesday, Brian transported all elective surgical cases in his Alfa Romeo Giulietta down to Limpsfield, operated all day Wednesday and hospitalised the dogs until they were fully recovered and had their stitches removed. If he performed an emergency operation at Pont Street, a ruptured spleen for example, he took that dog home with him that evening, and his Surrey RANA nursed it back to health.

Pet owners never saw the pain their dogs experienced after surgery. It took me some time before I fully questioned what I'd been taught, and started to use painkillers during and after not just surgery but any event that was potentially painful. When a canine parvovirus that caused acute gastroenteritis suddenly appeared nine years later, it was the dogs treated with painkillers together with more conventional treatment for serious gastroenteritis that were most likely to survive.

'She's walking on her own,' Pat reports on Monday afternoon.

'She went down the steps into the garden on her own,' Pat reports on Tuesday morning.

'She gave one of her toys a shake this morning,' I'm told on Wednesday.

Isn't it spectacular how dogs just get on with getting better, even after such pain and trauma? It impresses me as much today as it did then.

I had arranged to visit Bianca at lunchtime on the Wednesday, but ops took longer than expected and the afternoon was filled with appointments. I promised a quick visit to the nearby Wilton Arms, also on Kinnerton Street, to do a post-op check on their two cats I'd spayed on the Monday, so I asked Jane to rearrange the home visit for between 7.30 and 8 pm. After a pint with the publican, it wasn't until just before nine that I got to Bianca's sky blue painted terrace home off the Kings Road.

It is only when she answers the doorbell that I realise just how deliciously tall Felicity is, my height in her stockinged feet. In a short, dark skirt her legs are as long as Twiggy's but her curves are pure Italian movie star.

'Darling Vet. You're such a sweet man to visit,' she says, louder than I expect and kisses me on my lips.

'It's Bruce,' I say.

'Come in. Meet my friend Barbara. Stay. Have a drink? Have something to eat. Bianca is a miracle. A miracle! That fucking bastard Alsatian! I'll kill him if I see him again. I'll fucking castrate his owner. My husband will see to that. You've had such a busy day. I'm famished. Come in. Meet Barbara.'

Felicity's eyes are extraordinarily beautiful, their aquamarine sparkle enhanced by pinhead-sized pupils.

'Hi, I'm Barbara.'

Felicity's friend, a fringed willowy brunette in matching white top and hot pants, offers her hand then kisses me on both cheeks.

'Look at Bianca. It's as if nothing's happened to her. Isn't she marvellous?'

Bianca is resting alertly on a white leather sofa, and I go over and sit down beside her. She flinches and pulls away as I reach out to touch her.

'Hello, little girly. You're quite a tough nut, aren't you?' I say and offer her a finger to sniff, and she does.

For most operations, the surgical site is shaved. We used a noisy electric Oster clipper followed by a men's razor at Pont Street, but I'd worried that clipped hair might get inside Bianca's chest so I'd just scissored away the long white hair from the edges of her wound. Once I'd sewn the skin back together, there wasn't much sign of the trauma she had suffered. With her white hair covering her wound, I couldn't even see her skin stitches.

'What's her appetite like?' I ask.

'She adores prawn cocktails,' says Felicity, as she offers me a glass of red wine, spilling some as she fills my glass. 'Oh, fuck. Do you adore prawn cocktails? You must be starving. I'm starving. You must eat. You must.'

'Thanks, I'm okay,' I reply.

'No, you must. We're going to Annabel's. Please come. It's my thank you for what you did for Bianca. You must.'

Barbara adds, 'Do come. It's much more comfortable having dinner with a man.'

'Are you sure you're happy to leave Bianca alone?' I ask.

I can see that Bianca could safely be left but am looking for a reason to avoid 'socialising with clients', especially a married one.

'Of course she is! Thanks to you!'

'Will your husband join us?' I ask.

'Our husbands are shooting in Italy,' Barbara replies.

'Or something,' adds Felicity.

'I'm almost ready,' Felicity tells Barbara, and she leaves the room, only to return a few minutes later. Her long blonde hair, parted on the left and previously in a ponytail, now flows over her shoulders. Her platform heels make her tower over me. The only likeness between Felicity and me is our similar age and language. Otherwise we are from different leagues and hers is a lot more professional than mine.

I worked in San Francisco in 1968, at a hippy vet's clinic on Haight near Ashbury. Mort, my boss, would offer me a joint each lunchtime, and each lunchtime I refused with a 'Thanks, Mort. I don't smoke. Asthma.' One evening, after dinner with two friends, Jinny his wife provided us with just-baked brownies for dessert.

'Hash brownies,' Mort explained after I'd eaten three of them. 'Specially for non-smokers.'

That evening Mort and his friends minutely examined his Navaho woven-container collection.

'Wow, look at that!' Mort pronounced. 'There's a diamond-back rattler crawling around this one.'

I took the container in my hands.

'No, Mort. That's dark, dyed grass geometrically woven at a perfect 45-degree angle to make a symmetrical diamond pattern.'

I was too uptight to be affected, even by the concentrated THC drug in hash, but became familiar with its physiological effect.

Here in London's Belgravia, looking into Felicity's beautiful but now bloodshot eyes, I know that she is blown away on an industrial amount of it.

A Bentley car and driver mysteriously arrive outside her home and takes us to Berkeley Square. I am taken first upstairs to the Clermont Club, where Felicity and Barbara kiss seemingly everyone, then down a flight of stairs to Annabel's for dinner.

The staff know both of them and we're greeted with genuine smiles. There's a table waiting and we sit down and drink.

Then order. Then drink more. And eat. And we talk non-stop, but it's so loud in the restaurant I don't know if what I'm saying has anything to do with what Felicity is saying. I don't mind because I'm having fun and I have two stunning women for company

'Let's dance,' Felicity says to me between the main course and dessert and we do. She is a hugger. My love life is parched, but she is married and I am, you know, a Canadian.

When we return to the table, Barbara unexpectedly announces, 'Felicity. Must go. I have a doctor's appointment first thing tomorrow.'

She kisses Felicity goodbye and I see her lips say, 'Don't overdo it.' Barbara kisses me goodbye and leaves, and we return to the dance floor.

'Bruce is my vet. He saved Bianca's life,' Felicity says to a couple she obviously knows.

'Hello!' they greet me in unison, then continue dancing. Everyone seems to know Felicity, and their ease at seeing her with a man who is not her husband makes me feel more relaxed.

It is now after 1 am. I've always envied people who can live for the moment. I couldn't then and still find it hard to do. As I've mentioned, Brian had told me not to socialise with his clients. And this one is married. I explain to Felicity that I have to be at work in a few hours and she gathers up her things.

The doorman hails us a cab and Felicity tells the driver to take us to her address and then 14 Pont Street. As soon as the cab pulls away, without a word she leans over and kisses me – passionately. *Nice.*

We drive around Berkeley Square.

She hold my hand and places it on her breast. *Very nice.*

The cab drives down Piccadilly, through the tunnel under Hyde Park Corner, past Harrods and down Beauchamp Place, and we keep kissing.

Then Felicity takes my hand from her breast and guides it to her knee and along her thigh onto velvet skin. She is wearing garter and stockings.

Our kissing becomes more ardent and she moves my hand further. *When did you manage to rearrange everything that way?* But then it dawns on me, *No, it's not rearranged! Felicity, do you know that between there and there your knickers have no knickers?*

'You have reached your destination,' the cabbie announces.

Maybe not, but we are parked outside Felicity's home and we both sit back in our seats.

She opens her handbag and gives me a crisp £20 note.

'Pay the cabbie when he drops you home,' she says, then, 'Mmmmm' and gives me a last long kiss and leaves the cab.

'Got anything smaller?' the cabbie asks when we arrive at Pont Street and I proffer the £20 note. I think, *I have now*, but don't say it. When I see Felicity the following week, to remove Bianca's stitches, I give her a £20 note and explain she had given me too much for the cab. Felicity has no recollection of giving me the money but from the look in her eyes remembers the rest of the evening. Bianca still doesn't want me to touch her.

I ask Christopher when he next visits with a litter of Pekingese pups if he knows of the Templeton-Ellises.

'Felicity Templeton-Ellis is very alluring,' I remark casually.

'She may be moreish but avoid her with a barge pole,' he cautions. 'It doesn't matter how charming she is, he's ex-SAS and provides mercenaries for African dictators. Mostly former Foreign Legionnaires. His best friend Lord Lucan has just separated from his wife. They're both heavy gamblers at the Clermont Club. Ruthless. Completely ruthless. Brian pales into insignificance in comparison.'

'You're comparing Brian with the SAS?' I ask incredulously.

'Aren't you as frightened of Brian as I am?'

I say that I am intimidated by Brian but also see that he behaves as he does because he exemplifies the reserved Englishman.

'There's someone inside who wants to get out and have fun,' I remark.

'Well, all I see is a perfectionist who frankly I find quite scary,' Christopher says. 'And what's scarier is that tomorrow I have to take one of these bloody Pekes on a Swissair flight to Geneva, and I hate flying!'

'Okay, Christopher,' I reply. 'I have two questions: why don't you like flying and do people actually pay your airfare for you to personally deliver pups to exotic places – because if they do, I want to swap jobs with you.'

'I hate flying because I feel claustrophobic in planes, and yes, we provide a door-to-door service if that's what our customers want. This one here?' and he lifts the pup in his left hand. 'I'm delivering it to Yul Brynner in France next Friday.'

'Right then, the pub after work? I've got more questions and I owe you.'

We meet as arranged at 7 pm at the Nag's Head.

'There's a charity gala event in Belgrave Square this evening and I'm taking my girlfriend to it. British Red Cross. So just one drink,' Christopher explains.

Inside it is heaving as always, so once more we take our drinks outside.

'Do you seriously hate flying?' I ask.

'Everything about it. Going to Piccadilly to buy the bloody ticket. Checking in at BEA in Victoria. The coach trip to Heathrow. Walking across the tarmac. Climbing those rickety stairs. Finding myself incarcerated in a sardine can without a bloody can opener. Going through bloody Customs. Filling in the bloody tax forms because I'm importing goods. The bloody French. I hate it all.'

'So why don't you have one of your shop or kennel staff do the deliveries?'

'Because our customers want mother to deliver their pups, and if it's not mother then it's me. That litter of Pekes I brought in today? Royalty. Singlewell Pekes. And royalty have their own chauffeurs. The mother of that litter was a debutante at last year's Crufts. Are you going to Crufts? Dog royalty. You should. It's not simply a dog show, it's the start of the London Season.'

'The London Season?' I quiz.

'Bruce, you must go. It's the doggy equivalent to the Debutantes' Ball. Bossy women and moustachioed men. Only those with aristocratic credentials – they've won best in their class – are eligible to attend. Fresh-faced virgins displayed not just to eligible bachelors but to professional seducers. Parents choosing who will mate with whom. Stagey pomp. The participants all nervously eyeing each other. It's absolutely hideous and wonderful all at the same time.'

'But you said it's the start of the London Season. What's that?' I ask.

'Bruce, to understand the British you need to know what makes us tick. I'm sure just as I do you meet some wonderful people, but we also meet people who are utter snobs, who go to events because it's what aristos have always done. Go to Crufts. You'll see more ex-Colonial officers and their wives and retired colonels and their wives than anywhere else in Britain, unless of course you follow them through the London Season, to the Boat Race between Oxford and Cambridge on the Thames, then the Summer Exhibition at the Royal Academy and the Chelsea Flower Show, Trooping the Colour, racing at Royal Ascot, the Proms at the Royal Albert Hall and if you are willing to move up the Thames a little, to the Henley Regatta.'

Christopher laughs. 'Do you think they see the irony of an aristocratic event sponsored by Pedigree Chum?'

Before I can get a word in, Christopher adds, 'Listen, Bruce, must leave. That Peke pup I'm delivering to Yul Brynner on Friday? I'm taking my girlfriend with me. He lives at Le Manoir de Criqueboeuf about ten miles from Deauville. He's always sending us photos of his Pekes with his children. We've sold three to him. I've booked a hotel for Susannah and me in Deauville for the weekend, and I'm hoping we might be invited to his chateau for a meal. I'm picking her up now, then we're off to the Red Cross fundraiser in Belgrave Square. Why not grab a girl and join us there? But not Felicity Templeton-Ellis.'

Grab a girl? That was like, 'Why don't you fly to the moon?'

I did wander over to Belgrave Square. It's minutes from Kinnerton Street. The railings around the gardens had just been replaced. They were removed during World War II when the gardens were used as an Army vehicle compound. I felt out of place, on my own. I looked for Christopher, but in the thick crowd didn't see him. An artist, Feliks Topolski, was sketching people, with his fees going to the Red Cross. I sat for a sketch. Seventy-five pounds. Almost four weeks' salary. Still have it.

5

It was July and London was sunny, although the mood in the country sure wasn't. I was on a decent salary for the British, £21 a week when the basic wage was £11. But dock workers had called a national strike and the Queen, who had been visiting Canada, signed a State of Emergency within ten minutes of landing back in London.

There was a surly feeling in London. Lots of talk of 'us' and 'them', lots of national strife, but even so this was the best time ever to be a vet. That's because my profession was on a cusp. I was trained as an animal mechanic, but I already had a hunch I should be more than that. The equipment at my disposal was just starting to improve in capability. We were about to be the first clinic in London with an electrocardiogram (ECG) machine, although that depended on the strike ending and supplies coming through the ports once more. There were a few specialists around, but a vet like me was still a jack of all trades, expected to handle any animal emergency. I was able to do things my professional liability insurers would never let me do today.

'Bruce, St George's Hospital just rang. A horse has been injured by a lorry outside the hospital and needs help. Brian wants you to go.'

It is lunchtime and I am reading the ECG section of *Canine Cardiology*, one of the American textbooks I brought with me to London.

'Do you know how bad it is?' I ask Pat.

'The horse is standing and has a large flesh wound to its shoulder. That's all I know. It's probably one of Lilo Blum's. Her stables are in Grosvenor Crescent Mews.'

'Does Brian know I'm allergic to horses?' There's a hesitation in my voice.

'You mean you don't like treating horses?' Pat queries.

'No, I mean I'm *allergic* to horses. They make me seize up.'

'How did you get through college, then?' she asks.

'With friends covering for me.'

'Don't forget the bute. It's in the fridge,' Pat reminds me.

I packed my medical bag with Betadine,* a new skin antiseptic we had just purchased, developed by NASA for the recent lunar landings, xylocaine cartridges and the cartridge gun, a spool of autoclaved surgical silk ready for use, a selection of sterilised surgical needles, a surgical pack of forceps, needle holder, scalpel, scissors and swabs, the phenylbutazone, or bute, a painkiller and ACP, a sedative, in case the horse was difficult to manage.

'Did the knife-sharpener sharpen all the scalpel blades and scissors?' I ask.

'Yes,' says Pat, 'and Mr Singleton has ordered new, disposable blades, so we'll be hearing less bloody grinding from that sodding cart in the future.'

At a brisk walk in a fresh autumn wind it took less than five minutes to get to St George's, where the injured horse was standing on the crescent-shaped ambulance entrance,

---

* A brand of povidone-iodine.

surrounded by a crowd. There were several girls in nurses uniform in the throng. All of them looked gorgeous, even the ones who probably weren't.

A ginger-bearded man, blue-green eyes, my height – a little over six feet tall – and my age – late twenties – wearing an olive-green tweed hacking jacket, tan riding breeches and brown boots, was holding the reins and halter. He looked great. I was envious.

'Hi, I'm Bruce Fogle, the vet. How's the horse?' It is a little Arab-Welsh grey pony.

'I'm Jeremy Livingston and this is Euripides. He's surprisingly relaxed considering what has happened to him. I ride Euripides at lunchtime each day. He's immune to the traffic but today, as we turned into Hyde Park Corner towards the park, for no reason at all he came to a full stop. He has never done that before. The traffic stopped, but then a lorry tried to go around us and caught him on his port side. It looks rather angry, and so am I.'

By now, between working at the zoo and for Brian, I had been in London for almost a year, was getting more familiar with British understatement, and I liked it. It sat well with how I felt. I walked around to Euripides' left side and saw the damage, a raw, ragged skin tear about fifteen inches long, with many red trails of both dripping and drying blood running down his leg. Fortunately, there was minimal muscle damage under it.

'Nasty,' I say to the rider. 'Jeremy, are you his owner?'

'Yes. I stable him at Lilo Blum's.'

'Do you have your own vet?'

'Yes, Mr Eaton. In Sutton.'

'Before anything else, I want to give Euripides some painkiller,' I say. I get the bute from my bag, raise his right jugular vein and inject a few millilitres of it.

'Is Mr Eaton on his way?' I ask.

'I have had people ring from the hospital but they can't get hold of him. Will you please take care of the wound?'

'Yes, of course,' I say.

So far so good. In a horse stables, thanks to my allergy my lungs would have sounded like bagpipes by now, but outdoors at Hyde Park Corner they produce no whistles and breathing is easy.

Euripides is an experienced urban pony, wonderfully relaxed, so I don't use the ACP sedative. Pat's grinning advice as I left the surgery – 'If the horse is a male and you use ACP, remember you'll probably have to carry his penis back slung over your shoulder' – influences my decision to avoid it. ACP relaxes the muscles that keep a horse's penis where a horse penis should stay.

While Jeremy holds Euripides by his halter, I cleanse the tear with Betadine. On the upper edge of the laceration, one region of skin is raised and rounded. I feel both sides of the mass and it's as if a pellet has lodged just under the skin. I squirt xylocaine over the open flesh, then inject the surrounding skin, including on the far side of the pellet. On dogs I usually use about half a cartridge of xylocaine. Euripides needs six cartridges.

'How old is Euripides?' I ask.

'Fifteen this month.'

The hundred-yard spool of sterilised surgical silk is in a separate autoclaved bag, but as I open it the spool unexpectedly rolls out, not onto relatively clean pavement but into Euripides' fresh green manure. I am surrounded by a crowd of onlookers. I've dropped my suture material in horse poo. Can you imagine how I feel?

'Damn!' I mutter under my breath, but before I even think of asking someone to go back to Pont Street for more, one of the pretty nurses steps forward and says, 'Would you like me to get you some suture material?'

'If you could, that would be great.'

'What size?' she asks and I tell her '2–0', a size I feel comfortable with.

'Thank you so much. I'm Jeremy and this is Mr Fogle,' the rider says to the nurse.

'Hi, I'm Nicole,' she replies with such cute dimples in such rosy, soft cheeks that I forget about Euripides. I hadn't been on a date since I started working at Pont Street. My last date was with an American girl whom I met while working at the zoo. She'd come over to talk while I was examining a rhea, a South American ostrich-like bird that had a lolly stick stuck in its mouth, and asked me out. When she kissed me goodbye the following morning she said, 'You're cute. You're fun, but you need to be more assertive. If you don't ask, you don't get.' (*But I did get*, I thought at the time.)

Minutes later, desirable, shiny-haired, well-formed Nicole is back.

'This is what we use,' she says, and hands me a packet labelled 'Dexon'. 'It's absorbable, with swaged needles.'*

Nicole strips open the outer packaging and inside is further packaging. When I tear this open there is twelve inches of suture material, with a small, attached needle. I grasp the needle with my needle holders and push it through the horse's skin. It feels like putting a warm knife in soft butter – no resistance at all, and Euripides doesn't flinch. Using mattress sutures, each package of Dexon stitches no more than three inches, but Nicole is there, smiling, radiating hormone, peeling open the outer packaging each time she sees I need more material.

'If it's okay with you, I'm going to remove that little pellet of

---

* A swaged needle is attached to suture material without the need of an eye to thread the suture material through. It can also be called an atraumatic needle.

skin at the edge of the tear,' I tell Jeremy. 'I think it's a skin melanoma.'

'That sound's bad!' he says.

'Not as bad as they are in us. Melanomas are pretty common in grey horses as they get older. Usually around the bum. If you see one and it's easy to remove, it's best to remove it.'

'Would you like some formalin?' Nicole asks.

'Yes, please, if you have any,' and she asks one of the other nurses to get some while she continues to hand me more Dexon. Her hands are perfection. I continue to tidy the edges of the wound and place tension-bearing mattress sutures.

'Under the circumstances, your horse has a good name,' I comment to Jeremy as I place more stitches.

'Why is that?' he asks.

'Well, your horse gets back to his stables, the Italian groom goes over to sponge him down, looks at his shoulder and says, "Euripides?"'

I'm still the smart alec.

'Rather good that,' Jeremy replies.

In less than fifteen minutes, the wound is closed and Euripides looks rather good too. And my lungs are still clear.

'That's wonderful suture material,' I say to Nicole as I pack away my instruments. 'I'll tell my boss about it.'

'The surgeons here are always opening the outers but not using it,' she says. 'I'm supposed to throw it out, but that's such a waste so I keep it. The material is still sterile inside the inner packaging. I've got hundreds of packets. Do you want some?'

I want to say, 'I want some of you.' But instead I say, 'Yes, please,' and Nicole disappears through the emergency entrance to St George's. I decide that when she returns, I'll ask her out.

'That was excellent work, Bruce. I very much appreciate what you have done for Euripides. Will you walk with us back to the stables?'

'Yes, but the nurse is getting something,' and as I speak, delectable Nicole returns through the hospital door with a shopping bag bulging with Dexon packets.

'Nicole, I don't know how I could have managed without you,' chirps Jeremy. 'You are Euripides' guardian angel. If you are free this evening, would you like to join me for a glass of champagne at the Grenadier?'

Before I can say anything, Nicole accepts smooth Jeremy's invitation. I envy his utter ease with women. After a few more thank yous to those who had helped, Jeremy, Euripides and I walk up the mews by the side of the hospital to the stables.

'Jeremy, I've learned something today,' I say as we arrive and one of the stable cats comes over to greet us.

What I want to say is, 'What I've learned is that my last date was right. I have to be more assertive, like you,' but I find that too difficult. I find talking about feelings or emotions too difficult. I still do. That might be why I feel so comfortable with animals. We intuitively understand each other's feelings without having to put them into words.

'What I've learned,' I say, 'is that I'm allergic to horses in their stables but seem to cope pretty well if they're in fresh air.'

'Why not go riding, then?' Jeremy suggests. 'You might get less sensitive to them. Miss Blum charges £2 an hour, and now that you know him you can ride Euripides if you like.'

'I might just do that,' I reply.

And do something about my appearance too, I think but don't say.

6

I would like to think that my life is my own creation, but of course it's not. Our past lives on in us, integrated into our present, knotted so perfectly that sometimes it can be hard to know one from the other. All of us are built out of a succession of personal stories. I know my early experiences and my family's stories intimately but I don't know Brenda's or Jane's, so when I look at people like them I see unique, stand-alone individuals. They seem spontaneous. And somehow that makes me envious of them.

'You have *how many* cats?' I ask Brenda. '*Nine?* Do you know that's enough for a baseball team!'

Brenda, our trainee RANA, is orderly and fastidious, a tidy, proficient girl who always had everything – sedative injections, anaesthetic-filled syringes, surgical instrument packs, gauze swabs, suturing material – neatly laid out in perfectly straight rows for each surgical procedure.

I use the word 'girl' intentionally. Pat was in her forties, wise, experienced and reliable for advice. She instinctively knew where a conversation was going, and if it was going where it might get uncomfortable she gently guided it towards a better place. Today, her gift would be called 'emotional intelligence'. Pat was the surgery's unpaid counsellor, offering sound advice to the other staff and to me. I wonder if she realised that was her greatest strength. Whether she did or didn't, Pat was a grown-up.

So was Pat's assistant, Jane. In her late twenties, frumpy, with short hair that looked like she cut it with bandage scissors, thick, putty thighs and skin that went scarlet for no reason at all, Jane was a bit dull but steadfast. She was sober, sombre, married and, although she hadn't yet told us, pregnant.

Brenda was neat and petite, with green eyes, freckles that melded into each other and hair as shining red as an Irish setter's. She looked like the resolute, toothy-faced little sister of your best friend, and from my perspective someone who would never think of sex let alone have it.

She was concerned about one of her cats. 'I had four until yesterday, but the stray I took in last month? The one they found in the theatre foyer in Sloane Square? She gave birth last night and there's something wrong. None of her kittens are taking milk. I've got them in the incubator downstairs.'

We spiral down the stairs from the second floor flat we use as our lunch room during the day and where I slept at night, past the consulting rooms on the first floor and reception on the ground floor to a tall cupboard in the basement, where washed dogs are placed on wire shelves to dry after bathing. A loud hot-air fan at the bottom of the cupboard provides heat, and this is also the 'incubator', the environment where we can ensure added warmth for our patients.

I take out the wire cat carrier the litter is in, open it on the prep table and lift a kitten from the bed inside. It looks both right and wrong. It is plump and fleshy, but its head, rather than sitting between its forepaws, bobs too much and twists oddly. I hand the kitten to Brenda and examine the next. It looks better, but when Brenda puts the first kitten on a towel it starts to roll off it. When I place the second kitten on the towel it too rolls. So do the other three kittens in the litter.

In the meantime, their mother lies in her bed and contentedly purrs, looking relaxed as we take her kittens away from her. I squeeze her nearest visible teat, then another. Milk expresses easily. She has a good milk supply, has released it and the kittens look healthy but aren't suckling.

'Do I know her?' I ask.

'No, I told you about her,' Brenda replies. 'She's a stray, not a feral. She's lived with people. That's why I took her home. When the theatre manager brought her in, all she wanted was cuddles. I figured she'd be okay with my other three but never thought she was pregnant.'

Back in those days, vets saw cats to sterilise them when they were young or to put them down at the end of their lives, but rarely in between. We supplied flea powders for cats that went outdoors and now had a new, more effective organophosphate aerosol flea spray, although it was proving almost impossible to use because to a cat the aerosol sounded like another cat hissing at it. That proved fortunate for cats, as organophosphates were eventually banned because of their toxicity. Cats were very much second-class pets. Stray cats lived everywhere, from Belgravia coal cellars to Buckingham Palace's gardens, but especially in the many World War II bombsites that still filled London. Some of the grand terraces around Regent's Park and the whole south side of Fitzroy Square had not yet been cleared: perfect homes for rats and mice, and cats. Cats cost nothing to replace and there was always a ready supply of them. Taking them to the vet didn't offer good value for money, even if a consultation at the most expensive surgery in London, Pont Street, was two guineas including any injections.

But there was a new and promotable reason to take your cat to the vet. A vaccine had been developed to protect cats from a common, life-threatening virus called panleukopenia or 'feline enteritis', and clients were starting to bring their cats in for inoculations, as they did their dogs. The first vaccine was a modified live virus, changed just enough to stimulate protection but not cause disease in the injected cat. It was marketed by several vaccine manufacturers. More recently, a killed virus vaccine had become available. We used the new killed vaccine at Pont Street.

'Brenda, it looks like the mother either contracted feline enteritis virus during the first three weeks she was pregnant or she was vaccinated with live enteritis vaccine during those first few weeks, but either way the virus has affected the kittens' brains and they can't balance themselves. That's why they're not suckling. I'm afraid it's hopeless.'

Brenda had returned the kittens to their mother in her bed in the wire carrier. She reaches in and rubs the back of her fingers over them.

'They look so normal,' she says, and continues to gently stroke the litter. 'Why is it hopeless?'

'Remember your anatomy? The cerebral cortex for cognitive abilities and the cerebellum for motor activity? The panleuko-penia virus prevented their cerebellums from developing. It's hopeless because they don't even have the part of the brain they need for balance and coordination. That's why they roll on the towel. They can't tell up from down.' I look at this soft mass of innocence. 'And never will.'

The mother cat continues purring. She shows no resentment to our handling her kittens; she isn't protective, as a feral cat would be. She seems almost indifferent to them, as if somehow she understands they are not right. Brenda picks up one and thoroughly examines it, its closed eyes, its tight shut ears, and when her finger examines the kitten's mouth the tiny creature instinctively sticks out its thin, rounded pink tongue to suckle on it. Brenda continues examining the kitten, its drying umbilical cord, its belly, its bottom, then she puts her baby finger back at the tip of the kitten's mouth and once more the kitten tries to suckle.

She gently puts the kitten back into the carrier, but this time she puts the kitten's head close to the teat I had easily expressed milk from and holds it there. The kitten grasps the teat and sucks. Brenda takes her hand away, and as soon as she does the kitten rolls off the nipple. She picks it up, puts it back, and it latches on once more. This time she holds it there. And as long as she does, it suckles.

'It's not hopeless,' she says intensely. 'They can eat if I hold them while they suckle.'

'Yes, they can,' I answer. 'But what then? How do they live with half their brains missing after they finish suckling? How do they walk? Or groom themselves?'

Brenda continues to look at the kittens, not at me.

'I'm due my annual two weeks' holiday,' she says. 'I'm going to take it now.' Then she looks at me. 'Or is it better that I tell Pat I'm ill?'

'Brenda,' I said quietly, 'nothing can save them. It will be so much worse for you to have to put them down when they're bigger and you've put so much time into them. It's really best that I do it now.'

She looks intently at the litter.

'No,' she says after a long pause. 'It's not best.' I look at Brenda, this little tomboy in a trainee RANA's uniform, and see there is no point in trying to convince her she is wrong. I know she will regret her decision.

'Okay,' I say, 'we both go to Pat and tell her why you won't be here.'

'Bruce, did you have a rough weekend?' Pat asks when, three weeks later, she arrives for work on the Monday morning.

'What? Oh, no, I'm just growing a beard.'

'Whatever for? You're already handsome as you are.'

'And look fourteen,' I answer. 'Even you told me so. Girls aren't going to take me seriously if I look like their kid brother. And my clothes. Everyone's in velvet jackets and flowery shirts. I stick out like a hick.'

'I don't mean your beard. You look like you've got a hangover.'

'Oh, that,' I mumble. 'It's not a hangover. I've been helping Brenda feed the kittens. Thank goodness it's every three hours now and we sleep holding them so they don't roll all over the place.'

'*We* sleep with them?' Pat comments, her eyes twinkling.

Brenda had taken me seriously without my having to grow a beard, but I was not sleeping with her. I had been going over to her place in Battersea every spare evening after work to help her with the kittens, and our relationship was relaxed but remained platonic.

'We take turns feeding them, then both of us hold the kittens in our hands in a normal position for an hour or so before returning them to their mother. Separately. We do it separately. I'm just helping out.'

'Hmmm,' Pat replies. 'It's a busy morning but not much surgery so far. Mr Singleton is at the Royal College and you're seeing the Hoechst rep at lunchtime. Oh, and Professor Levene's secretary at the Royal Marsden called to thank you for that horse tumour you dropped off for him. It was a melanoma.'

After removing the small growth from the grey pony outside St George's Hospital, Brian had told me to take it over to the Royal Marsden Hospital on Brompton Road and leave it for Arnold Levene.

'Levene's a rare find,' Brian had explained. 'He has an unquenchable appetite for information. We send all our tumours to him. I heard about him from Jean Shanks.'

Dr Jean Shanks, a clinical pathologist, owned Jean Shanks Laboratory on Harley Street. We looked after her dog and sent all our blood samples to her human lab for analysis. It would be another few years before veterinary clinical pathology labs became common.

That morning I saw my first case of 'old dog encephalitis'. The mature black Labrador's nose looked like dry, browned cauliflower. So did the thickened pads on his paws. His dark stained teeth were cracked and broken, with large pits of missing enamel. I saw at least one dog like Scamp every week, survivors of distemper infection. The changes to their pads and nose leather gave the infection its common name at that time, 'hardpad'.

Scamp's damaged teeth told me he had probably been infected with distemper while he still had his baby teeth. Just as using the antibiotic oxytetracycline in pups results in their adult teeth erupting stained bright yellow, infection with distemper virus as a pup results in the adult teeth erupting with badly damaged enamel. That's if the pup survives its distemper infection. Most don't.

Scamp was eight years old and apart from the looks of his nose, teeth and foot pads, he had no other sequels to his infection, not even muscle tremors. He had been healthy for years, but now his owners say he is constantly circling or walking into the corner of a room and pressing his head against the wall as if he were trying to relieve an enormous migraine.

'We know what it is,' his owners tell me, 'and we don't want him to suffer, so we've brought him to be put down.'

I didn't argue. It doesn't take long in veterinary practice to understand that there is such a thing as a good death. This would be an easy one. More difficult are those that leap on you unexpected, that involve pain or suffering. My baptism was a Yorkshire terrier puppy, screaming in pain after having her head crushed. The damage was so extensive I could see bits of skull bone embedded in her brain. I felt unbearably helpless and thought if that's how I feel, can you imagine how the pup's owner feels? Sure, it's another species. Pets are not our children but we raise them, feed them, care for them, often sleep with them. Can you imagine how vulnerable an owner feels when her pet is in obvious, excruciating pain and there's nothing she can do about it? But I can do something. I can kill that pet quickly and painlessly. And as horrific as that sounds, that's also a good death.

Jane raises a vein in Scamp's front leg and I inject a lethal dose of pentobarbitone.* His heart stops beating in less than a minute and he dies.

'May I send him up to the college?' I ask his owners. 'They're doing a study on old dog distemper there.'

'Yes, if it helps,' I'm told, and as soon as his owners leave, Jane and I carry Scamp's body down the two flights of stairs to the prep room where it is left on the treatment table.

Brian returned at lunchtime and came downstairs to see what had been booked in, in his absence. Nothing today, and I explained I'd put down the dog because of old dog encephalitis and was harvesting Scamp's brain for the distemper study at the Royal Veterinary College.

'Send the owners a letter with your condolences, on headed notepaper. Write it yourself. Don't type it. They'll appreciate your sympathy.'

At that time we post-mortemed just about every animal that died. There was and still is no better way to know how disease progresses or what has caused death or disability. These days it

---

* Pentobarbitone is an anaesthetic now rarely used for anaesthesia. I used a modification of pentobarb called thiopentone routinely for general anaesthesia.

is different. I am rarely given permission to carry out an autopsy. People are more squeamish and feel there is a sanctity in the body of their dead pet. People want their pets buried or cremated without the physical body having been 'abused' by knife, scissors or bone cutters.

Abdominal and chest post-mortems are relatively easy to cut open and sew shut. Not so brain PMs. The skin has to be cut and parted, then muscles removed until the bony junction between the skull and the atlas, the top vertebra, is exposed. Then the top of the skull is removed with bone cutters, much like opening a trap door. When it goes smoothly and everything gets neatly sewn back in place once the brain has been removed, it is, in an aesthetic sense, just fine. Today, the bone in Scamp's skull is yielding reluctantly to the scissors-like cutters. It is messy and takes longer than expected. The drug company rep from Hoechst has arrived and I have asked Pat to have him wait in my consulting room, but she replies that he wouldn't mind seeing a Labrador with its brain being removed so he joins us in the prep room.

'Johnson,' he says. 'How are you?'

'Bruce,' I reply. 'Fine, thanks. Sorry if I can't shake hands. Is Pat getting you a tea?'

'No, Sir. I've asked Pat to wait until you can join me.'

I am supposed to be concentrating on cutting off the top of Scamp's skull but can't take my eyes off Johnson's black leather shoes. They're five-eyelet Oxfords buffed so brilliantly they shine like mirrors.

'I'm impressed,' I say. 'I was once a sleeping-car porter for Canadian Pacific Railways but I was never able to get shoes to shine the way you do.'

'RAF,' Johnson replies. 'I was a police dog handler until I left. I would like to be a full-time dog trainer, but there's simply not a sufficient demand.'

Before coming to London, I had seen the RAF Police Dog Team put on a show of their dogs' skills at the Royal Agricultural Winter Show in Toronto. German Shepherd dogs obeying commands, attacking baddies, jumping through fiery hoops. It was all very impressive.

'Why did you leave the RAF?' I ask, and Johnson tells me the police dog training centre had moved to Essex, and Essex wasn't for him.

'How do you do it?' I ask, about his shiny shoes, not dog training.

'Yellow duster, high-wax boot polish, water, elbow grease, beeswax.'

He looks at my feet. Having dropped wearing sandals, I am now wearing a pair of brown slip-on penny loafers with dimes inserted in their top pockets. They very much need a shine.

'In your business, you might want to just give them a good application of brown shoe wax, a proper brushing, then apply clear floor polish. I'd suggest Johnsons.'

There is mischief in his eyes and I develop an instant liking for the man. Although we share pints at the Nag's Head over the two years I remain at Pont Street and I go to one of his evening dog training classes a few weeks later in Maida Vale, I never ask Johnson's first name. He never offers it.

Pat calls downstairs that the body man has arrived. With Scamp's brain in a glass jar of formalin, I ask Jane to sew up his scalp skin, let me know when she has finished and I'll help her put his body in a hessian sack, ready for the body man to pick up. I stay out of the way when the knackerman comes in his filthy brown overall, trailing the smell of death. I once saw him throw the hessian body bags in the back of his truck, then unwrap a sandwich from its wax paper and eat it. Without washing. With massive black flies surrounding him. At that time I didn't know that the body man collected for renderers, who supplied rendered agricultural animals to pet food companies for tinned dog and cat food. I knew that cats were collected for their skins. I was told they were shipped to Poland and turned into gloves. It didn't enter my mind that the pet food my patients ate might include rendered dog and cat.

Johnson has booked a visit because he wants to convince us to switch from the dog vaccine we are using, Burroughs Wellcome Epivax, to his company's vaccine Maxavac. He has two trump cards. If we use his vaccine, he will supply us with ongoing disposable needles and syringes. We can retire the glass syringes. Even better, his vaccine is in rubber-topped vials. I'll never cut my fingers again from sawing, and breaking in half, those glass vials.

'What about "blue eye"?' I ask.

Preventative dog vaccination was and still is a profound life saver. But those first vaccines could cause problems. I had read that some live distemper vaccines could revert to infectious forms and cause lethal brain inflammation – encephalitis, like Scamp suffered from, but within months of an inoculation rather than years after infection. I knew that the hepatitis component of the vaccine I was using caused 'blue eye' in some dogs, a fluid swelling or oedema to their corneas. With most dogs the corneal oedema lasts no more than two weeks, but for some dogs the condition lasts longer or is complicated by ulcers.

'We use a slightly different virus in our vaccine,' Johnson explains. 'CAV-2 rather than CAV-1. It is CAV-1 vaccines that cause blue eye.'

'And encephalitis?' I ask.

'We use the Onderstepoort strain of distemper virus in Maxivac and are confident it cannot cause post vaccinal encephalitis. Dr Fogle, you are obviously knowledgeable and interested in the science of vaccines. I've invited several London vets out for early drinks this evening. Mr Singleton tells me he'll be taking calls this evening. Would you care to join us?'

I hadn't asked anything remotely scientific but liked being told I was knowledgeable. I wondered why Brian would be taking calls but not enough to see that evening drinks had in fact been engineered by him.

'Where and when?' I ask.

I arrive at the basement bar in the Nag's Head on the dot at 7.30 pm. The room is even smaller than upstairs, low ceilinged, narrow and with an inviting coal fire on the back wall. It is late autumn and the nights have closed in. The temperature has suddenly dropped into the 40s, not cold by what I am used to, but in London's damp climate it feels bone-chillingly bitter. I am happy to see the roaring fire in the fireplace, with Johnson and three other men standing in front of it.

'Dr Fogle, what would you like to drink?' Johnson asks.

'Bruce. Call me Bruce. A Guinness, thanks.'

I have no appreciation of warm English beer and prefer a cold pilsner, but have developed a fondness for the burnt flavour of a creamy-headed dark Guinness, especially on a cold evening in as inviting a pub as the Nag's Head. The others are drinking English beer, except the oldest, who has a Scotch in his hand.

'Do you know each other?'

'Hi, Keith, John, Mike,' I say to the three vets I know, then turn to a new face, a round-headed, round-eyed older man with curly dark hair that is just starting to fade away. I can see it will eventually make an early exit from his head.

'Bruce, meet Frank Manolson. He's a fellow Canadian of yours. And a wonderful writer. His surgery is on the Kings Road.'

'What the fuck are you drinking?' Frank asks as we are introduced.

I've mentioned I was raised in an extended family that never swore. I really didn't hear swearing as part of normal conversation until I moved to London. Frank's language offends my ear but there is no attitude in his voice, certainly no anger or condescension. There is surprise, an almost innocent incredulity. '*What on earth are you drinking?*'

'Come with me,' Frank says and we walk over to the bar.

'A J&B, barman,' he says, and when it is poured we walk back to the vets around the crackling fire. 'Have that, then your stout.'

Keith, Mike, John, Frank and I talk about cases, about difficult clients but mostly about Brian, whom they respect a lot, as I do, but are also intimidated by, as I am.

'He's asked us to form an emergency night and weekend rota,' Keith casually mentions to me.

'Yes, that's one of the reasons we're here,' Johnson adds. 'Mr Singleton asked me to be an independent arbiter in case you want to ask an outsider what he thinks.'

'Well, as you're here, what do you think?' I ask, and Johnson says he can see no possible reason why we don't form a rota.

'My clients won't come back when they see the fucking facilities the rest of you have,' Frank says.

'Swings and roundabouts, Dr Manolson,' Johnson says. 'I suspect it will all average out.'

'It's too far for my clients to travel. Halfway across London,' adds John, whose surgery is in Holland Park. 'I can't see it working. I appreciate Brian asking me, but I'll opt out.'

Johnson turns to Keith. 'Mr Singleton tells me you take each other's calls when needed, so I imagine you're in?'

Keith puffs on his cigar and nods in the affirmative.

'And you, Mr Gordon?'

Mike also nods his approval.

'Dr Manolson?'

'I'll have to think about it,' he replies. 'Let's have another drink.' We go for another J&B and Guinness, and when we return to the roaring fire we both sit on the same small side table.

'When did you graduate, Frank?' I ask.

'Fifty-one,' he answers.

'And how did you end up on the Kings Road?'

'I was meshuganah,' he answers. 'I sure as fuck wasn't going home.'

'Where's home?' I counter.

'A hundred miles outside Medicine Hat. Arse end of nowhere. Would you live in a got farlazn place like that?'

'*Meshuganah. Got farlazn*. Frank, are you Jewish?' I ask.

'Fucking right,' he replies. 'Ham on rye Jew. Same as you.'

I smile at his accuracy. 'So how did you graduate from Guelph in '51? They didn't accept Jews until 1960.'

'The registrar was a sodding bugger. On my application, for Religion I wrote "Cattle". He saw my address was the Circle M Ranch. It never entered the bastard's mind that a cattle rancher was a bloody Jew.'

Sodding. Bugger. Bloody. Frank may be a fellow Canadian but he was swearing like a Brit.

'Did you come here from Guelph?' I ask.

'Via Rome,' he says. 'I worked for the Food and Agriculture Organisation before I came here. That's how I became a writer. I couldn't find a job when I got here. Thought I'd be a small animal vet but couldn't remember a damn thing about dogs, so I made an alphabetical list of what I thought I'd need to know. Abscess. Boil. Canker. Distemper. Turned it into a book, *D is for Dog*. It sold well and Pelham the publishers wanted another, so I wrote *C is for Cat*. Now I'm writing a sex book. *My Cats in Love*. Have another drink.'

'At Guelph, I edited the university newspaper,' I tell Frank. 'I'd love to write.'

'Money for old rope,' he says. 'Pour yourself a drink. Hit the keys. Don't forget your carbon paper. Get a damned good editor. Everyone thinks you're fucking brilliant.'

'So the rota,' I continue. 'If you're in, we've got enough vets for Monday to Thursday. That means you're on call one night a week and one long weekend a month. You know I won't steal your clients.'

'I trust the others, but you're a landsman. Can I trust a shmuck like you?'

'What do you think?' I say to him. He doesn't answer that but instead says, 'Why are you working for Brian?'

'He offered me a job and Jim Archibald told me it would be good for me to make my mistakes thousands of miles from home.'

Frank puts his arm around my shoulder and puts his head close to mine. I can see in his eyes that he's had several J&Bs before I arrived.

'You need to visit my surgery to see how much fun you can have. I need a good vet. Come and visit.'

7

The buzzer on my phone rang.

'Mrs Wax is here,' Brenda says.

Frank was an okay guy. He was foul mouthed, but I instantly liked him. Mrs Wax was something else. The ECG machine had arrived and we became the first surgery in London to have such equipment. She had returned with Mitzi, saw Brian, who admitted the dog, and I carried out the ECG by pushing reusable stainless steel needles through Mitzi's skin just above her elbows and hocks, attaching the ECG's clamps to the sticking-out sharp ends of the needles. I had never done an ECG before, so my ability to interpret the results was abysmal. These days, I use electrode jelly and gentle skin clamps and have a cardiologist interpret the results. At Brian's I was willing to, *wanted* to, try everything. What experience gives you is not just a more realistic idea of what your limitations are but the realisation that doing very little, often nothing, provides the best outcome. But in Mitzi's circumstances, doing nothing would lead to early heart failure. Medicines to help her heart would prolong her active life.

The client day sheet in front of me says that Mrs Wax is bringing in Trixie, one of her other Miniature Poodles, and when she enters the consulting room she and Trixie are accompanied by another slightly larger black Poodle. Mrs Wax is smiling.

'Ah, Dr Fogle. Mr Singleton explained that you're a *Doctor*. I didn't know that you are a *Doctor*. I thought you were a *Mister*.'

I smile back but offer no explanation for why I can be called 'Doctor'.

'Good to see you. How's Mitzi?'

'Wonderful, wonderful. But I'm here for Trixie. She is ready for breeding but the stud,' and she looks with dismay at the larger Poodle, 'he won't perform. I've massaged him but he refuses.'

In my first months at Brian's, I'd learned to ask, not to tell.

'And Trixie's ready?'

'Oh, yes,' Mrs Wax says. 'She'll stand for the postman.'

'And how can I help?' I ask.

'I want you to artificially inseminate her,' she replies in a very matter-of-fact way, as if this were a technique I was familiar with. 'That's why I've brought along Mr Spot.' She turns to the male. 'Mr Spot! Sit!' and he does. 'He's very obedient. He'll do anything you ask him.'

I don't have any idea what to do, but I say, 'Mrs Wax, leave them with me. I'll collect semen from him at lunchtime and do the AI.'

'I know he's in good hands,' she replies, and I wonder whether behind her helmet of hair there lurks an ironic sense of humour.

After morning appointments finish, I go downstairs where Pat, who is theatre nurse that day, has already taken a vaginal smear from Trixie and has a glass slide under the microscope waiting for me to have a look.

'She's ready,' Pat says, as I look at the smear.

'You've had a look?' I ask.

In veterinary practice people may book appointments to see a vet but spend as much or more time before and after their appointments with the clinic's staff, RANAs as they were then, or RVNs, Registered Veterinary Nurses, as they are today. For me, working with a really good nurse was – and still is – better than working with a really good vet. It's not just that nurses have a complementary range of clinical abilities but that they also intuitively interact with clients in a more natural way. They often know more about clients than vets do.

'Yup,' Pat answers. I look down the microscope eyepiece and see, as Pat had seen, that all the vaginal wall cells are large and angular, with nuclei so small they are virtually invisible. If Trixie were earlier in her season, I would be seeing smaller, rounder cells with very visible nuclei.

'Mrs Wax might be tricky but she's an experienced breeder and knows when her dogs are ready to mate. Trixie's ready, so he's the problem.'

'Now the fun begins,' Pat says. 'Who has the honours?'

'I'll do it,' I say. 'And we need a container.'

Pat hands me a half-pint beer mug.

'Are you a left-handed or right-handed wanker?' she asks.

'The last time I wanked anything was a Saanen goat at college,' I reply. At college, my best friend and classmate, Ian, lived locally and I often had dinner with his family. His father was professor of obstetrics and reproduction, so I was the student he easily recognised when in fourth year we were introduced to AI techniques in livestock.

'Fogle. Collect a semen sample from that goat,' Prof. Barker snapped at me as he handed me an artificial vagina. One farm hand held a tease goat steady while another walked an excited, prancing white billy goat down the barn hall towards her. As he started to mount her I grabbed the goat's penis, but before I could get it in the artificial vagina he ejaculated, shooting me in my eye. Prof. Barker thought it was very funny as I wiped dripping semen off my cheek with the arm of my lab coat. So did the rest of my classmates. No matter how much I scrubbed, the smell lingered on my face for days.

Pat rubs a gauze swab over Trixie's vulva and puts it under Mr Spot's nose. His ears perk forward. I kneel on the dog's right-hand side with my left hand free for wanking and the beer mug in my right hand. Turns out I'm a left-handed wanker.

'Ready?' I ask.

'He's ready,' Pat says, and with Pat gently preventing him from walking I massage the prepuce, his foreskin, and feel the middle of his penis, the 'bulbus glandis', swell. That's the part that enlarges when dogs mate. It prevents the male from withdrawing after he ejaculates. That, in turn, prevents other dogs from immediately mating with her.

When the swelling is firm I retract his prepuce, grab his penis and with my rubber-gloved hand keep massaging. Mr Spot starts to thrust his pelvis. He is deadly serious. No sense of humour. I look over him to Pat, who is grinning. In her ill-fitting dark green uniform with its silly white apron, married to I don't know who, she's never mentioned, her hair too curly and coloured, her arms too mottled and fleshy, Pat was sexless, but when she smiles, and she often does, she has the most alluring dimples. They are so deep they cast shadows on her cheeks.

'Pat, don't say a thing!' I say sternly.

'I can tell you're experienced at this,' she says.

I continue massaging Mr Spot's penis, then as his thrusts slow and reach their climax, I bend his penis downward, squeeze the apex with my thumb and forefinger, and he ejaculates several millilitres of crystal clear fluid followed by a few more millilitres of greyish-white liquid into the beer mug. His semen keeps flowing, the last quantity as clear as the first.

'Good dog!' Pat proclaims, gives him a hug and puts him in a kennel. 'And if you behave yourself, Dr Fogle will be very nice to you again.'

I swirl the semen in the beer mug until all three different colours are thoroughly mixed to a uniform grey-white, warm a glass slide under hot water, draw a drop out with a sterile syringe, place it on the slide, cover it with a coverslip and look at it under the microscope. The sperm look textbook perfect, virtually all of them actively wriggling.

'Okay, lift her bum off the floor,' I tell Pat, and she lifts Trixie's hindquarters up at a 45-degree angle and places the dog's head between her knees.

'There's no dignity in this,' Pat says.

'You mean there's dignity in normal sex?' I ask, and we both smile.

I stroke the dog's vulva. It's called feathering and at that time vets thought that it helped stimulate semen transport once the semen is inside. It doesn't.

'Have you ever been to Raymond's Revue Bar?' Pat asks.

I don't answer. This is the hard part and I am concentrating.

I clean the region and insert a urinary catheter into her vulva.

'Mr Singleton uses a plastic drinking straw,' Pat tells me when I ask her to get me a catheter.

'Too blunt for me,' I explain.

But I am inserting blind and the catheter is small enough to go through the urethra, rather than the cervix, and if that happens I'd be inseminating her bladder. I gently push the catheter forward. If it is in the thin-walled bladder, I'll be able to feel the tip by palpating the back part of her abdomen, and I can't feel it, so I draw semen from the beer mug into a glass syringe, attach the syringe to the catheter and gently squirt the fresh semen in.

'Keep her hind raised for fifteen minutes,' I tell Pat.

'Whatever for?' she says and puts her down. 'If it's going to work, it's going to work. You don't need gravity to get pregnant,' and she leads Trixie to another kennel, then telephones Mrs Wax to tell her the dogs are ready to be collected.

'Can you imagine what Mrs Wax will be like if this doesn't work?' Pat says.

'You're the grown-up here,' I say. 'I'm off on visits. When she picks up the dogs tell her the vaginal smear was good, so were the sperm, but with AI it's a 50:50 chance of pregnancy. Book an appointment for a little over three weeks.'

That evening after I finished work, I walked down to Sloane Square and hopped on a bus that took me down the Kings Road, past Peter Jones, Cecil Gee (where I'd just bought myself some trendier clothes), Royal Avenue and the Chelsea Drugstore, the Markham Arms where I thought the most stunning mini-skirted girls, meeting their lanky-haired, frilly-shirted, gormless boyfriends, hung out, the fire hall, the ambulance station, Mr Freedom and Granny Takes a Trip, then the World's End pub, where the bus continued into a part of London I hadn't ever visited, the Fulham end of Kings Road, where I was having dinner with Frank Manolson.

Frank's surgery was in a row of small, low-built, two-storey shops on the north side of the road. It was easy to see the surgery had been converted from a terrace house, with two rooms on each of the ground and first floors, a 'two-up, two-down'. It was almost 8 pm but the waiting room brimmed with pet owners and pets. There was no staff member to tell I'd arrived so I nodded a hello to some of the people in the room and stood by the door. Soon, the door to the back room opened and a couple in their late fifties, both with heads bowed, emerged, silently walked through the waiting room and out the door. Frank saw me through the open door and without saying anything waved me in.

'Never know what shit is gonna happen,' he says as he washes his hands. A small girl in her early twenties, with short, straight mousy hair, smiling eyes and lips like Mick Jagger's, is putting the body of a small, fat, black and white short-haired dog in a hessian sack. She ties the sack with string and carries it out a door into a yard, adding it to several other hessian sacks.

'I sit here all day with fuck-all to do, and come six o'clock everyone decides to go to the vet's.'

Frank doesn't offer appointments. In a working-class part of London, a vet's surgery is unusual. He charges eight shillings, that's 40 pence, for a visit, plus injections and tablets.

He goes to the door to the waiting room. 'Next, please!' he says, and his clients know their order of arrival and enter his examination room in correct sequence. There is a dog with large, bleeding tumours around its anus. Frank gives it a pen-strep antibiotic injection, his nurse collects ten shillings from the owner and arranges for the dog to come back the following day for another injection.

The next dog is vomiting. Frank gives it two injections, the sedative ACP and a vitamin B12.

At Brian's, clients get monthly invoices and pay by cheque. Brian has a bookkeeper. Frank has a jam jar. He collects twelve shillings, putting the money in the jar on a side table.

They are told to come back tomorrow if the vomiting continues. The next patient is an elderly cat, no muscle, just hanging skin, with thick, crusty discharge glueing its eyes shut.

'I'm sorry but there isn't anything that I can do,' Frank tells the cat's owners, and I can see genuine concern – empathy – in Frank's eyes.

'I know, Vet,' the cat's owner, another woman in her late fifties, says.

'Will you bury her?' Frank asks.

'I live in a flat,' she answers.

'You can leave her here,' he replies, as he injects lethal pentobarb directly through the chest wall into the cat's heart.

'How much is that?' she asks. He answers, 'Half a crown.' She hands a ten shilling note to Frank, four times the cost of the euthanasia and says, 'Give the rest to charity.' He puts his thick arm around her shoulder. 'You did the right thing. When you think you're ready for another cat, let me know. Don't go to Club Row. I'll be able to find you a healthy local kitten.'

There are nine dogs and cats in his waiting room when I arrive, even though surgery hours finished at 7 pm, and Frank efficiently works his way through all of them in less than forty-five minutes, including a litter of Jack Russell pups brought in for their tails to be docked.

'You know how we did this on my ranch?' he smilingly asks the pups' owner. 'With our teeth!' he laughs. 'You can feel exactly where to do it.'

Frank doesn't use his teeth. He uses a set of heavy nail clippers, crushing the tail then twirling it clockwise until the rotations cause the tail to drop off in his hand.

Every patient gets an antibiotic injection or a B12 injection. The only one that doesn't is the Jack Russell mother. That evening most dogs go home with tablets or capsules that Frank dispenses. The Jack Russell mum goes home with sterilised bone flour to add to her food.

After his last patient leaves, Frank turns to his assistant. 'Leave the floors until tomorrow,' he says. 'You've been a good girl. Thanks for staying late.' And she smiles, disappears upstairs, comes down a few minutes later, now in bell-bottoms, platform shoes and a frilly white shirt, throws on her coat, says, 'Bye' and is out the door.

She transforms herself from nothing to someone I would be much more interested to spend the evening with than old Frank.

He locks the front door behind her.

'I'll show you around,' he says. 'We do everything here,' he explains, and I can see that his examination table doubles as his prep and operating table. A wheeled ether anaesthetic machine is sitting in the corner of the room.

'The privy's attached to the house and I converted that to kennels. I put in a toilet upstairs. Here's the pharmacy,' and he opens a cupboard filled with large brown glass jars of white pills, red pills and green capsules. There are ten bottles of vitamin B12.

'Why so much B12?' I ask.

'People don't expect to pay for bullshit. They pay their good money for stuff. Everything gets a B12 injection and everything gets pills or capsules. That makes them feel they've got something from their visit.'

'What are the pills?' I ask.

'Starch. Placebo pills. They're made for us but are just as handy for dogs. Now then, before we have dinner, let's have a drink,' he says and I follow him upstairs, where there is a sitting room including a kitchenette, a bedroom and the small washroom he mentioned. He pours me a large Crown Royal whisky.

'The one thing these fuckers don't understand is good rye,' he says, as he drains his glass then takes off his shirt to change into a fresh one.

I notice abrasions down his side.

'What happened?' I ask, nodding towards the dramatic scabs on his shoulder and back.

'Oh, that,' he answers in a matter-of-fact way. 'See that fire escape over there?' and he directs his eyes to a thick rope on a red reel attached to the wall beside the single front window overlooking the Kings Road. 'I was having a drink last week with a couple of guys I know and I'd just had that fire escape put in, and we decided to try it out.'

'How does it work?' I ask.

'Nu-Swift come over, measure everything, then instal that reel. If there's a fire, you clamp that ring round your crotch and waist, and exit through the window. It lowers you a foot a second to the ground and there's another loop ready to lower the next person, until everyone's out.'

'But how did you get those abrasions?'

'You know how fucking filthy it is out there, so before I jumped out the window I stripped off. Didn't know I'd bounce against the wall on the way down.'

After another large rye, it is into Frank's Rover P5 saloon and a five-minute drive to the Great American Disaster on Fulham Road.

'Anyone else coming?' I ask.

'My wife's at home. Somerset,' Frank says.

'I thought you lived in London?'

'Got property all over Fulham, but I can tell you one plain fact, Bruce. You can't graze Shorthorns on Eel Brook Common.'

There is a line of Americans waiting outside the restaurant, but Frank walks past them into the inviting warmth.

'Frank! Great to see you. Give me a few minutes and I'll get you a table,' the man at the door says.

'Alsatians,' Frank whispers.

We sit down, order beers and burgers with the works, then Frank turns to me.

'Should we join the EEC?' he asks.

'Yes, sure, why not,' I say. 'I like the idea of no currency control when I go to France.'

'Ken Tynan says the EEC is the most blatant historical vulgarity since the Thousand-Year Reich.'

'What? He's comparing an economic community to the Nazis?'

'Okay, forget that,' Frank says. 'A guy got hit by a car outside the surgery yesterday.'

'What happened?' I ask.

'I took a couple of towels and went out to see how he was. He was groaning, so I put the towels under his head and said, "Are you comfortable?" and he said, "I make a living."'

I smile. 'Okay. So we come from the same place,' I respond and Frank nods an acknowledgement.

'An Englishman, a Frenchman, a German and a Jew go walking in the desert and get lost,' I say. 'They run out of food and water. They're dying of thirst. The Englishman says, "I must have tea." The Frenchman says, "I must have wine." The German says, "I must have beer." And the Jew says, "I must have diabetes."'

Frank smiles. 'Heard it before,' he says. 'Why did Moishe's dog eat the leg of the table?' and before I can answer, Frank does. 'Because he was Chewish,' then he continues. 'We've both heard all of them. No farting around. Come work for me. You know those fuckers where you are, those nasal bastards with their expensive gun dogs and their heads up their own arses hate us. You saw tonight I see real people with real problems. Come work with me.'

I knew Frank wanted me to work for him, but I wasn't prepared for such a forthright offer. I liked him, even with his foul mouth and heavy drinking, but his clinic was minuscule, his treatments dreadful and, well, he was foul mouthed and drank heavily.

'Bruce, do you know what a house off Wandsworth Bridge Road costs? Five, six, seven grand tops. In Chelsea it's thirty thou and no change. Minimum. Brian's clients would rather die than live with my customers in Fulham.

'Work for me and you'll have your own home. I'll make a thousand quid down payment and pay you fifteen hundred. It's a cash business and you'll get another twenty quid a week, tax free. Think about it.'

We eat our burgers. Delicious burgers.

'And what's with the facial hair?' he says. 'You fucking look like Jesus.'

8

'Fogle, we are going to inspect Grace's ovaries later this morning,' Mr Hime told me as I arrived at the zoo hospital. Like Brian, Malcolm also used the plural 'we' to keep an emotional distance from what he did.

'That's dramatic!' I replied.

Grace was one of the Bengal tigers, the smallest of the females at the zoo. The Zoological Society of London (ZSL) had a tiger-breeding programme. Grace hadn't come into season for two years and Malcolm Hime, the Brylcreemed, rodent-nosed Chief Veterinary Officer wanted to find out why. This was exciting, although it hadn't been in my plans. Then again, becoming a vet hadn't been in my plans. I am a vet by accident. Almost everything in my early life was by accident. I was latent. Reactive. When my mother visited the high school principal because of her worries about the academic progress of my older brother Robert, the principal told her that Robert wasn't her problem, I was.

'Bruce is a dreamer. He knows he can get by without doing anything and he's happy with that.'

Choosing to study veterinary medicine was an accident, not a plan. On the Fogle side of my family, no one had ever gone to university. My father was a florist, my grandfather a tailor and

my great, great-great and great-great-great grandfathers black-
smiths. My Fogle aunts, Nettie, Jeannie, Edie and Mary, with
their fine leather gloves and veiled hats and tweed suits and
neatly crossed legs and Glaswegian accents, were more Scottish
than Jewish. My father's religion was fishing and although I
didn't have a serious conversation with him until he was into
his nineties, one thing I knew as a teenager, without him telling
me so, was that he expected me to marry a Jewish girl.

My mother's brothers were all university graduates, many in
medicine. My best friends were Breslin cousins and my closest
cousin, Calvin, had decided to study veterinary medicine. When
Frank Manolson told me I was a 'ham-on-rye' Jew, he hit the
bull's-eye. On my way to Hebrew School on Tuesdays and
Thursdays, I stopped off at Calvin's for his mother to make me
a bacon and egg sandwich. Although my culture was Jewish, by
the time I was a teenager I knew I didn't believe in a pre-
destinationist god. My mother's father, a dairy farmer, was the
first in his family not to study as a rabbi but only because his
father had emigrated from Europe and his son had to earn a
living in the New World. An unwanted marriage had been
planned for him and he hightailed it from Rochester, New York,
across the border to the emptiness of Canada. His sons, my
uncles, amused me with stories of milking their cows then
lowering the churns into the well to keep them cool until they
were raised and taken by horse-drawn cart to the milk train
heading to Toronto. But with my tall, ramrod-erect, remote
paternal grandmother as my only living grandparent, with no
one in my extended family speaking English with any foreign
accent other than Scottish and living outside of the communi-
ties with large Jewish populations, I didn't feel 'as Jewish' as I
felt my classmates at Hebrew School were. That may be a
reason why I felt comfortable with the idea of becoming a vet,
rather than the prototypical doctor or lawyer.

Just before the Ontario Veterinary College's first term was due to begin, Calvin withdrew and switched to human medicine and with my typical latency I didn't, so I found myself in Guelph, treading water. With only a few exceptions I found the school, my classmates and my classes boring, so I gravitated to the arts side of campus and got involved with the university newspaper, *The Ontarion*, writing for it and editing it one term. Academically, I did what I always did, I got by, until in second year I failed my anatomy exam by one percentage point and was kicked out of the university.

'That's what happens when you write those terrible editorials criticising the administration,' my mother shouted at me in exasperation. 'You think they couldn't find an extra percentage point if they liked you?' I never told her that those lucid and opinionated editorials were written by my classmate, Ian, the son of the obstetrics and reproduction professor, but signed by me.

For a month after I was expelled, I sat in my parents' home doing nothing, then one day I decided I had to show them what a mistake they'd made. I decided to get a job at the veterinary college, get to know the faculty and hope they might help. I worked for a year at the Virus Research Institute, and its Director John Ditchfield and the Head of Pathology Jim Schroeder petitioned the Senate to allow me to return, but something else happened. Working in research, following the trail of a germ that turned out to be an influenza A virus, tracing the travels of that virus to southwestern Ontario, where it suddenly killed almost 100,000 turkeys (and in doing so killed itself off because it no longer had turkeys to infect), back to Connecticut and Massachusetts, with tangents to common terns in Scotland and turkeys in South Africa, and finally back to its source in Petaluma, California, injecting embryonated hens eggs, titrating solutions, doing haemagglutination inhibition tests, performing post-mortems, attending weekly meetings – it all made veterinary medicine exciting, stimulating, worth doing. At first I wanted to get back on the course to show 'them' what a mistake they'd made. Now I wanted to get back because I actually wanted to get back, to become a vet, to engage in veterinary research.

My girlfriend, Andrea, was certainly happy to know I was there for another four years. My parents disapproved of her – her father might have been a Supreme Court judge but she wasn't Jewish – so we stayed at my parents' house, my house, only when they were away. They once arrived home unexpectedly. Andrea giggled a 'Hello' and thought it was quite funny. My mother told me never ever to use her house again for immoral purposes.

Andrea and I coordinated our summer jobs so that we were in the same locales, usually Guelph, but in 1967 we spent the summer in Ottawa, where she worked in the Department of Justice and I did research at the Food and Drug Directorate, part of the Department of Health. Then my brother got married and I was told I could not bring Andrea with me to the wedding. Even in a relatively secular family like mine, that was the reality of my adolescence and it was a factor in us eventually going our separate ways. That influenced my thoughts on where I wanted to work after graduating. I was keen to be 'somewhere else', not near home.

The associate dean of the college, Tom Hulland, had taken an interest in what I'd do after graduating, and found a possible job for me at Yale Medical School in New Haven, Connecticut, in immunopathology, the new discipline studying how the immune system goes wrong. I don't know why I said so, but I told him I'd prefer to first work in a zoo. It was a remarkably random thought I plucked from the ether. I can't remember ever wanting to *visit* Toronto Zoo let alone work there, and although

I'd visited Regent's Park Zoo in 1964 and San Diego Zoo in 1968, I hadn't bothered in either instance to investigate veterinary care or opportunities. Three weeks later, I had a travel scholarship to study the fatty acid profile of African herbivores in captivity at Regent's Park Zoo, and that's why I was now going to help Malcolm Hime investigate why the tiger hadn't shown signs of estrus.*

Malcolm was a quixotic man. I spent most of each morning in his office doing nothing, listening to his dreamy ideas about what the zoo should be doing. His knowledge, of research and researchers, was striking. When I had a question, he always had a detailed answer. Malcolm felt that the zoo was primarily a research institution and that visitors were at best a nuisance. When he introduced me to Sir Solly Zuckerman, the Secretary of the ZSL, and Michael Brambell, the Curator of Mammals, I learned they both agreed that this was the primary role of their zoo.

Working on the clinical side, I couldn't help but agree that visitors could be pests. At the zoo, the keepers were the equivalent of pet owners, and they called me to their enclosure when they anticipated or saw a problem. A visitor-induced problem might be as avoidable but as simple as the lolly stick stuck in the throat of a rhea (unlucky for the rhea but lucky for me, because at least it lead to a date), or as devastating as a rhinoceros death caused by a tennis ball tossed thoughtlessly into its pool and swallowed, causing a lethal obstruction discovered only on post-mortem. I am told this continues to be a common cause of death in captive rhinos today.

During the morning of the tiger op, I completed my clinical rounds. A crisis with a greater kudu took up much of my time.

---

* Estrus is the period of receptivity and fertility in females. For cats, usually when daylight is increasing.

The mother had stepped on her newborn calf, and the calf's plaintive cries had distressed its mother so much that she was not letting down her milk. I injected her with oxytocin* and half an hour later milked her to provide sustenance for the moribund calf. It died later from its abdominal injuries. In the meantime, the tiger's keepers had lured her into a large 'crush' crate, a metal crate with top and sides that could be moved inwards to immobilise the big cat in a fixed position. At 11 am Malcolm had given the cat a sedative at its enclosure, and by the time the trolley arrived at the operating room the cat was sedated, deeply enough for a trap door to be opened, a forelimb drawn through it and thiopentone anaesthetic given intravenously.

The surgical team, already dressed in white surgical gowns, watched as the crate was opened and the cat, weighing around 120 kilogrammes, was lifted by four keepers onto the operating table. Malcolm asked me to stretch her head forward and open her jaws while he deftly inserted an enormous endotracheal tube into her windpipe, inflated it and connected her to the inhalant anaesthetic, Penthrane, a variation of ether. She was rolled on her back, her abdomen shaved and scrubbed, and I went to the scrub sink and washed up, hoping I'd be allowed either to open or sew her up.

'Fogle, this is Whitehouse,' Malcolm says as I return, gloved and ready. 'Mr Whitehouse is going to demonstrate how he can inspect the reproductive tract without surgery.'

Mr Whitehouse was a gynaecologist, one of a string of many contacts Malcolm Hime had. 'Good morning, everyone,' Mr Whitehouse says. 'This is a laparoscope. I have never used it on a body quite as beautiful as this, but I hope to be able to visualise the ovaries and Fallopian tubes, and with Mr Hime's veter-

---

* Oxytocin is a naturally occurring hormone that is used to increase the strength of contractions in the uterus and thus speed up childbirth.

inary advice, determine whether there is a physical problem in these areas.'

With help from two surgical nurses he brought with him and listening to Malcolm Hime explain where things were in the tiger's belly, Mr Whitehouse made a small incision, inserted a tube into it and filled the cat's belly cavity with carbon dioxide. He made a second stab incision just below the cat's umbilicus, inserted his rigid laparoscope and, with his eye on the eyepiece, moved it around.

'This is the monopolar unit we use for tubal ligations in women. We're experimenting with a bipolar unit.'

'What's the difference?' I ask.

'Both ligate through electrocoagulation, but we think the bipolar one does so more accurately. I'm retiring this unit, which is why I'm happy to use it here today.'

The gynaecologist quickly found one of the tiger's ovaries and asked Malcolm and me if we'd like to have a look. Malcolm looked first, described it as normal, then I looked through the laparoscope. It felt like looking through a kaleidoscope but with a glistening grey ovary at the end. Each time Mr Whitehouse viewed a different area, he let us look.

When he had finished, I asked if I could have a general look inside the cat's abdomen, and he let me gently play with the scope, instructing me how to lift fat away to better see viscera.

After he finished his investigation, finding no physical abnormalities, the big cat, now off inhalation anaesthetic but still asleep, was transferred back into her crate and, accompanied by an oxygen cylinder feeding pure oxygen into her endotracheal tube, wheeled back to her enclosure. When her eyes began to blink, Malcolm deflated the enormous tube and withdrew it through her mouth. The front and side of the crate were both removed so that when she stood up she did so away from the exit to the outer enclosure.

Walking back to his office, Malcolm is pensive. 'Fogle, we're a primitive profession. We think we can do everything ourselves. Do you know there's not a single recognised consultant vet in the country? Thank goodness there are men like Whitehouse with their broad interest.'

That isn't exactly true. The very first veterinary 'specialists' are now working at the veterinary schools, but there are no formal means of recognising their skills. Who develops parameters for recognition? The Royal College of Veterinary Surgeons? The veterinary colleges? The British Veterinary Association? The British Small Animal Veterinary Association? Who takes charge? It's a muddle.

9

We love doing things our own way and always think our way is best, but if you are starting from fresh like I was – seeing an itchy cat or a coughing dog for the first time, meeting people who speak your language but don't use it the way you do – then you don't have your own ways yet. You're like an open container waiting to be filled. As a university student, I had my own political views and was dead happy to confront, to challenge, the views of the university administrators. I am, by nature, anti-authoritarian, although it wasn't until decades later that I thought about why I was and still am.

I now understand that I think the way I do because of my upbringing. When I wrote my first book, *Pets and their People*, ten years after the tiger op, and telephoned my mother to tell her it had received excellent reviews, she warmly congratulated me, told me how wonderful it was, then added, 'and remember, sonny, when you cook chicken soup, it's the scum that rises to the surface.' I share her radical distain for authority.

Thinking back, I was an irritating little fester. But curiously, I never challenged the veracity of what I was being taught by my teachers. We were told that all the screaming that dogs do when they recover from surgery wasn't pain. That was simply going through the excitement phase of coming out of anaesthesia. I believed that.

But now, six months into working for Brian, questions were seeping into my mind.

One thing was for sure. I was learning a new language. Fast. Not just different words, such as *boot* for trunk, *lorry* for truck or *bonnet* for hood. I was learning how to use words in an understated British way. *Mustn't grumble. Jolly good. Quite pretty. Not bad. Bit of a nuisance, that. Well done. Nice. Not very clever. Sorry.* I learned what *gobsmacked*, *skint* and *knackered* meant. But it was and is the British use of irony that I loved the most. I felt completely comfortable with it.

It wasn't ironic that I wasn't dating. I had my chances but the girls I was meeting at Pont Street, fabulous looking as they were, seemed out of my league. Keith, one of the vets I had met, called them Mayfair Mercs, on the prowl for their fortunes. That certainly excluded me and might be the reason why, when I finally met someone I felt comfortable dating, she came from my background.

Throughout November it constantly rained. Each morning, rain hammered against the window of my bedroom at Pont Street, scolding me about I don't know what. London was inside a permanent grey cloud. I knew that if I was in Ontario, I would need sunglasses to protect my eyes from the brilliant reflection off pristine snow. We Canadians are freshened by the sparkling colours of the seasons. The British are weathered by wind and rain. Now it was December, the last browned leaves were dropping from the London trees, the air was crisp and dry, and the sun was finally shining brilliantly from its southern horizon. So I walked up Sloane Street into Hyde Park, around the Serpentine to Marble Arch, to be entertained at Speakers' Corner.

As always there were a few dogs among the crowd, let out of their homes in the morning to do as they pleased during the day, then returning home in the evening. Most of these dogs learned to be streetwise, but not all of them were successful. At Brian's, we repaired a couple of bone fractures each week, almost all caused by road traffic accidents.

It isn't thronged as it is in warm weather, but the habitual speakers are there and each has his own crowd, listening, responding, heckling. I walk past a bearded regular in belted trench coat, standing on a short stepladder with his professionally painted sign, 'Holy Spirit Teaching Mission', at his feet. I am not interested in his literal interpretation of the Bible.

A man around my age, with Afro hair and a Jamaican accent, wearing a fitted, navy blue wool topcoat, is waving his arms as he speaks, and I walk over to listen. He is surrounded mostly by other Caribbean men.

'Is the Bible the word of God or of man? It is the word of Almighty God!' he thunders, answering his own question before any of his listeners can. I walk on, joining a small group listening to a middle-aged blonde woman with an East End accent.

'You'll regret it. You'll regret it! It's the bleedin' French what's behind it all. Bleedin' George Pompous-arse. We don't need no decimal coins.

'It's a conspiracy to make us all Europeans. Write to the Queen. Visit your MP. You can still stop it. You know why they really want to get rid of pounds, shillings and pence? It's so they can all put their prices up when they make us do decimal.'

'It's not the French, it's the Germans,' a listener shouts.

'We won the war. Why should we listen to them?' he continues.

'It's different now, mate,' another listener says. 'That Willy Brandt. He's okay, what with what he just done in Warsaw.'

'They're all bleedin' politicians!' someone else in the crowd shouts.

'Yes, but he meant it,' the second man replies. 'You can't fake that look on his face. A fucking German on his knees? That was spontaneous, mate. He meant it.'

I walk on to the next speaker, someone I recognise as a regular, with a lined and gaunt face, a balding head and thin, wispy
hair, a pencil-thin moustache, wearing a sheepskin overcoat,
standing on an upturned fruit box. In the group listening to him
is an attractive, short-haired brunette around my age, wearing
a mink jacket and accompanied by an Italian Greyhound wearing a grey wool sweater. The dog, the only one I see that day at
Speakers' Corner, stands silently by her side, his ears flattened
back against his head.

'You are wrong, my noble friend. And you are weak in spirit,
and that is why they have been able to control your life and the
lives of your antecedents,' the speaker says.

He continues, 'My simple but well-meaning friend.
Christianity was manufactured by Vatican Industries Ltd. It was
founded by Emperor Constantine and Sons in AD 325. It's a
business with guaranteed profits and limitless volunteers. The
Chairman of the Board is the Pope.'

The speaker speaks with the confidence that all regular
speakers have.

'Shame!' someone heckles from the crowd.

'If it's so profitable, how did the Jews let it slip from their
hands? They know where there's profit,' another heckles, and
there is an acknowledging murmur from the crowd.

'I would tell you, my learned friend, but there are spies here,'
the speaker warns.

'Why would spies come to Speakers' Corner?' another shouts,
and the crowd chuckles.

'To have a good time, just like you. Perhaps you're a spy,' the
speaker retorts.

'Don't fucking call me a spy!' the heckler shouts back, in
genuine anger, and all of us feel the tension rise.

'Take care, my friend,' the speaker counsels. 'If you are too
unruly, the police over there will put you in a cell where a twenty-

stone copper will accidentally fall on you. Don't you wish it was that lady copper?' and he turns his head towards two of the constables who regularly attend Speakers' Corner each Sunday.

His humour relieves the hostility.

I see the woman and her dog move on, and I follow them to listen to a young speaker I haven't seen before, younger than me, with a beard much like the one I now have, in jeans and a navy blue woollen donkey jacket with black leather shoulders..

'The Tories will bring back capital punishment and take away all the rights workers have died for. Heath is worse than Wilson and Wilson was a traitor to the cause. There is a conspiracy between them to prevent you from gaining your freedom. Only communism gives you freedom.'

'Wot? Like the freedom the bloody Czechs have?' a heckler remonstrates.

'Exactly what is communism?' another asks.

'Communism was created by Karl Marx to dethrone the right-wing capitalist bourgeoisie from their oppression of you, the people,' the young man replies.

'That's Groucho Marx,' someone shouts.

'Speaker, what does bourgeoisie mean?'

'It means you eat more than you can chew,' another listener replies.

'Karl Marx wrote *The Communist Manifesto* …' the speaker continues but he is shouted down with, 'That's the *Communist Fiasco*!'

Another listener joins in. 'You know why you're wrong?' and doesn't wait for the orator to answer. 'Because Karl Marx forgot about human nature.'

'And you are a capitalist pig!' the speaker replies, and I wonder why, if he is at Speakers' Corner, he says such a childish thing.

'And you are a communist monkey!' the heckler retorts. 'Has anyone got a banana for the monkey?'

'I'm no monkey!' the speaker shoots back. 'I've been to uni!'

'And what did you study there?' the same heckler asks. 'Philosophy? That's unlikely. Phartology? That's more like it.'

'I studied philosophy!' the speaker replies, with petulance in his voice.

'Can you pull your left ear?' his heckler asks.

'Why should I do that?' the now sloped-shouldered speaker responds.

'The toilet needs flushing,' his heckler says, and the crowd roars with laughter. The young man steps down from his box and I decide that if I speak to the girl, I won't tell her I've been to university.

I watch her stroke her dog's head, give him a treat from her jacket pocket and walk on to another speaker. I do too, and now stand beside her listening to a frumpy, high-pitched woman wearing a large CND button denounce America's involvement in Vietnam.

'The world's greatest superpower is killing or seriously maiming a thousand innocents every week in a tiny, backward nation. They are proud of what they are doing. Proud. They tell us they are saving the Vietnamese and the world from communism, and if Vietnam falls to the communists all the other Asian countries will follow like dominoes. Do you believe this?'

'No!' shout back several listeners.

'The war in Vietnam is a conspiracy of the military–industrial complex. It is war that drives the American economy. Americans think that war is good for them. Look at how they treat their Negroes. They did the same at My Lai. They don't care if they massacre yellow people.'

'That's not true!' the girl beside me shouts back. 'We care as much for yellow or Negro people as we do for anyone else, including you. There's a world struggle between totalitarianism and democracy. It's people my age, my friends, who are dying in Vietnam. We are willing to spill blood to defend you and your way of life.'

I am impressed by her confidence, and her willingness to take on the speaker.

'Miss, like so many of your countrymen you are what I call a provincial imperialist,' the polished speaker retorts. 'You only know your own history and are insensible to everything and everyone that is not part of your parochial atmosphere. You believe Senator McCarthy and J. Edgar Hoover because you have no concept of world history.'

'You have no right to criticise what we do without knowing all the facts,' the girl says.

'Do all the facts include what your government did to those opposed to the war at Kent State University? Do the facts include how your eminent paediatrician Benjamin Spock is vilified by the Nixon Administration? Do the facts include that your president lies to you to protect the military–industrial complex?'

'Well, he's a slime bucket but he's my slime bucket, and it should be left to me and my fellow Americans to criticise my government,' she says.

Listeners chuckle at her response.

I lean over closer to the girl. 'Terrific! You told him off. Are you visiting London?'

'Hi. No. I live here.' I can see she is livid with anger.

'I wish I could get my words out better,' she says. 'I hate the Republicans but you people paint all of us with the same brush. You don't know how hard it is to fight the Administration.'

'I'm not British,' I say.

'Oh. Yes. I wasn't listening,' and now she turns to me and relaxes.

'Hi. I'm Rose. Where are you from?'

'Hi. Bruce. From Canada.'

'Hi. I thought you were American. You have to say "oot" or "aboot" for me to hear you're Canadian. Are you visiting?'

'No. I live here too.'

'What brings you here?' she asks, and I explain the scholarship to Regent's Park Zoo followed by the job at Pont Street.

'That's a coincidence. That's where I take Bobby. To Mr Singleton.' Rose introduces me to Bobby, who shows a complete lack of interest in my touch or my words.

'And you?' I ask.

'To be honest, my parents arranged for me to be here to help get over a guy. I thought he was great and they didn't. I work at Sotheby's, and by the way, they were right. He wasn't.'

She didn't have to tell me that last bit, I think.

'Did you bring Bobby with you?' I ask.

'Oh, no. I'd never put a dog through a year of quarantine. I got him after I got a house.'

Own home. Minutes from where I work. Gorgeous face. Dog lover. Opinionated. Was it fate that brought me to Speakers' Corner today?

The morning's sharp sun gives way to a steel grey sky, and we talk and walk back through the park to Belgravia, stopping at the Nag's Head for a drink by the fire, and more talking. Rose hasn't been here before. She has to be home by 2 pm, she explains. She tells me she always calls her mother at that time, 9 am Boston time. I am enchanted. I ask her out for dinner the following evening.

Christmas is approaching. London is a mess. There's a council workers' strike, so garbage fills the streets, water supplies are threatened and Christmas has been called off. No Christmas lights! There's also a national power workers' strike and the government has invoked another State of Emergency. Can't these people sit down at a table and work out their problems?

Monday was another day of learning, unsettling, although it started brightly. The first client was the granddaughter of the Sultan of Johor. 'No touching,' Pat tells me and I don't understand why until I meet her, a supremely confident, long-haired, slim twenty-year-old, in hip-hugging, tight satin jeans and a transparent blouse. I meet beautiful women every day but she is meltingly eye-catching. Her smooth Chihuahua has itchy skin.

'If her grandfather is the Sultan, does she call her granny "Sultana"?' I jest with Pat after she has left.

'Yes,' Pat replies unexpectedly. 'But not the way you mean. A Sultan's wife is a *Sultanah*, with an "H".'

The rest of the morning's appointments were uneventful, but for one. Pat had booked in, as a courtesy consultation, the window cleaner's dog. The window cleaner, always accompanied by his male Collie-type dog Hamish, cleaned the floor-to-ceiling windows each Monday. Regardless of the weather, Hamish always lay on the pavement outside the clinic until Jock had finished, then jumped to his feet and accompanied him to his next shop.

'He's got no eenergie, Vet,' Jock explains, as best I can tell. Jock's working-class Glaswegian accent is almost impenetrable.

I look at Hamish's gums. They are pale. I listen to his heart. It sounds normal. I palpate his abdomen. It is pendulous and I feel a large mass, grapefruit-sized.

'Jock,' I say, 'I think he's got a mass in his belly and it's bleeding. I can have a look and see what I can do, but we have to be prepared for bad news.'

'Aye,' he says and this big man, this bull, gets down on his knees and looks straight into his dog's face. His dog stands motionless. Jock moves forward on his knees to be closer, gives his dog a hug then he stands up.

'Aye. Do your best.' As he passes me to leave the room he puts his hand on my shoulder, for only a second, and I feel his tight squeeze.

I know now how intense the attachment can be between people and their dogs, even if I didn't then.

Jane is surgical nurse, and we set up an intravenous saline drip, hanging the glass drip bottle from a drip stand. I inject fast-acting barbiturate, place an endotracheal tube down his windpipe and attach the breathing bag and tubing to the new halothane vaporiser. It was exasperating acquiring the equipment. I wasn't yet familiar with how passive business practices are in Britain. Brian had told me to research vaporisers and report back, but when I telephoned the distributor, BOC, the salesman said, 'You're a vet? What do you want a halothane vaporiser for?'

I fumed. 'Buddy, are you trying *not* to make a sale? What is it with you people!' and we got our equipment.

'Put bath towels on both sides,' I tell Jane, once she has Hamish scrubbed and on his back on the operating table. 'This may be messy.'

It is. Hamish's belly is filled with blood that has haemorrhaged from his spleen. I use the loud suction machine, but even so, blood overflows onto the surrounding towels when I cut open his belly. The bleeding tumour in his spleen that had felt grapefruit-sized, is in fact more the size of an orange. I lift the entire spleen out of Hamish's belly, lay it on top of him, clamp off all the arteries feeding the spleen, then the veins, then remove the entire organ. Once more, it isn't the first time I have removed a spleen. I had removed one during surgical exercises at college. This was my second.

With the spleen removed and the belly no longer filled with blood, I can now look at Hamish's other organs. I'd hoped the tumour was restricted to his spleen, but it isn't. There are small nodules throughout his liver. It is a metastatic tumour, one that has spread though his body.

'Damn!' I mutter.

'You did your best,' Jane says. 'Better to put him out of his misery now.' Jane is a sensible, pragmatic nurse.

'Ask Pat if we can get hold of Jock,' I tell Jane, and she leaves, returning with Pat.

'No, he's out working,' says Pat, 'and besides, he doesn't have a telephone at home. What have you found?' she asks.

'Haemangiosarcoma,' I answer. 'Spread to the liver.'

'Is the liver bleeding?' she asks.

'No. Not yet.'

'If you don't put him down, how long do you think he has to live?' she asks.

'I don't know. But it's maximum months, if not weeks.'

'Bruce, it's your decision what to do. You might want to know a little about Jock. His wife died of breast cancer around two years ago. His only son died in a road traffic accident last summer.'

Doing is the easy part of medicine. Deciding what to do is the toughest part. I look at Pat and know where she is taking me, and I am in a quandary. I am there to help animals, to alleviate their suffering. Now she is telling me that I should sew up Hamish, knowing he has untreatable cancer, for the sake of Hamish's owner. But I also know that this is exactly what my instincts are telling me, that I should commit this dog to a continuing decline because I don't know how to cope with kill-ing the last living member of Jock's immediate family.

I silently sew up Hamish.

'Give him lots of pethidine,' I tell Jane. I am now using that painkiller liberally. I have decided that what I was taught is wrong. When Jock returns at 6 pm, I explain to him that I have stopped the bleeding by removing the spleen and that Hamish will feel better for a while because he no longer has a blood-filled belly, and that his energy might increase for a while because his bone marrow can make new red blood cells but that the tumour has spread extensively to his liver and his remaining life will be short.

'Aye,' he says. 'I appreciate your honesty.' And he takes Hamish home.

That evening I met Rose as planned, for a drink at the Chelsea Drugstore on the Kings Road and then a meal at the Chelsea Stockpot. I tried to be but I wasn't much fun. During dinner she asked me if something was troubling me, and I told her about Jock and Hamish and how torn I was over who I was there for, the dog or his owner. After dinner I walked her back to her mews house off Belgrave Square, where she invited me in for a coffee. I stayed the night and wondered the next day whether she slept with me because she felt sorry for me. Bobby certainly didn't. He may have been barking instructions, but more likely was muttering expletives as he balanced on my back.

Why Rose? I was surrounded by 25 million British women but my first British girlfriend wasn't British. I think I know why. By the time we left the Nag's Head three hours after meeting in Hyde Park, I knew exactly who Rose was. She might be from Springfield, Massachusetts, 400 miles from where I was raised, but we shared an idealistic, liberal, educated North American background. At university both of us participated in civil rights organisations, me the local Student Nonviolent Coordinating Committee, or SNCC, and Rose the more radical Students for a Democratic Society, or SDS.

Rose was from a politically active family and her parents opposed her participation in the SDS. They refused to let her attend a teach-in at her university, but she did anyway. When she told me the novelist Norman Mailer was one of the speakers, I thought her parents were right to try to prevent her from going. I thought he was a self-serving blowhard.

A few years before the SDS teach-ins began, my family opposed my going to the American South with the SNCC's 1964 Freedom Summer, to help black Mississippians register to vote. I passed the SNCC's screening interview, quietly held in the coffee shop on campus. I think they were weeding out students with a 'white man's burden' complex. Looking back, I was almost comically the archetypal volunteer, a white, secular Jewish university student from the northeast United States or neighbouring Ontario and Quebec. Unlike tougher Rose, I caved in to my mother's pleas and instead got a summer job with Canadian Pacific Railway as a sleeping-car porter.

Rose went home a few weeks later for Christmas with her family, leaving Bobby with the Grievsons at Town & Country Dogs. They kennelled select dogs in their own home. The rota was working well and although Tuesday was my day, I volunteered to work on Christmas Day, a Friday, and was able to handle all the emergencies myself without having to call in Brenda, who had also volunteered to be available.

After the long Christmas break, it was back to the routine of work. The medical challenges I was confronted with each day were falling into a rhythm that I understood and expected: advice and inoculations for new pups, itchy skin, broken bones from road traffic accidents, spay and castration operations, vomiting, diarrhoea, distemper, training advice and the best part, the unexpected. I resumed my seven in the morning weekly riding lessons at Lilo Blum's stables, something I started in the previous autumn, riding Jeremy's Euripides. Perhaps it was winter when there are less allergens in the air, but it seemed to me I could stand in a stable with twenty steaming horses, bales of hay and insouciant stable cats and not seize up as I expected to.

'Bruce, be in my office in five minutes,' Brian says as I walk through the front door from my riding lesson. 'There's something I need to discuss with you.'

I go upstairs, quickly change from my riding clothes and meet him in his office.

'Mr Eaton has lodged a complaint,' he says.

'Who's Mr Eaton?' I ask.

'He's a colleague in Sutton. He says you operated on his horse without his permission.'

'His horse? It's not *his* horse. It's the owner's horse, Jeremy's horse.'

'Did you operate without his permission?' Brian asks.

'Wait a minute. Has he complained to the RCVS?'

'He tells me he hasn't yet contacted the College and I will ensure he does not, but before I ring him back I need to know the exact sequence of events. Did you try to contact him before operating on his horse?'

'I didn't. And it's not his horse. The owner did, or someone acting on his behalf,' I say. 'Does the owner know Mr Eaton is upset?'

In human medicine in the UK, medical doctors work in a culture where they don't criticise each other. Vets work in a different culture, a commercial one. Many think we're in competition with each other. Money is at stake. There's much less criticism today than when I started in practice. Now, it's more behind each other's backs. Then, the best way to criticise another vet was to report him to the disciplinary committee of the Royal College of Veterinary Surgeons.

'I don't know,' Brian says, 'and of course it is ludicrous for Mr Eaton to complain when you treated his patient in an emergency, but this is how some of our colleagues think. I need to know all the facts so that when I ring him back I can give him a stern bollocking for making such a frivolous complaint.'

Brian pauses and puts down the fountain pen he is taking notes with.

'Bruce, most of the complaints we receive at the College are like this. Not from the public. They are from fellow vets who need to be dragged into the twentieth century. Do you know if we have an address or telephone number for the owner?'

'Easy,' I reply. 'It's his horse I ride when I have my lessons at Lilo Blum's. I'll get it for you at lunchtime.'

Walking across the hallway to my consulting room, I wonder whether I'd have the same type of irritation if I worked for Frank. I haven't yet got back to him about his offer but think that as no private vets are particularly interested in looking after working-class pets, other than Frank or charities like the RSPCA and the Blue Cross, it might actually be less stressful working for him.

Rose had returned from Springfield on Sunday and picked up Bobby from Town & Country Dogs. This evening we have tickets to see a play, *Flint*, in Soho, and the day is filled with the rhythm of the January needs of London's dogs.

Puppies and kittens are popular Christmas gifts, so January should be a pleasurable time, watching cartoon innocents boldly investigate the consulting room floor, bounce like joyous springboks from person to person, thrive on the exhilaration of simply being alive, embark on the pleasures of life. In most instances this was true, but distemper was still the most common infectious disease I saw, and Christmas's presents now came in as January's tragedies.

'Where did you get him?' I ask when a couple from Pimlico put their sad Jack Russell pup on the examining table.

'The pet shop on Tachbrook Street,' they tell me. 'He's not eating. And he's sluggish.'

The pup has a fever and a snotty nose. His owner tells me he also has diarrhoea. Another distemper pup. I know he'll probably improve for a while, that his fever will subside and his appetite return but then, more likely than not, in a short while his brain will become inflamed. He'll become sensitive to light, or look like he has a searing headache, or drool saliva, or develop muscle twitches or have seizures. Most pups that develop some or all of these conditions are put down within a month.

Johnson, the Hoechst rep, sold us vials of Maxaglobin, a distemper antiserum. 'We have a dog colony in Germany,' he told me. 'We vaccinate them with our vaccine, then collect serum from them. That's why it's expensive.'

This pup hadn't yet developed pneumonia, the most common secondary bacterial infection, so I inject him with the new type of penicillin we have, ampicillin, inject distemper antiserum and arrange for him to be brought back at the end of the following day for continuing treatment.

The Sunday morning Club Row street market in Shoreditch in the East End of London was where most pet shops got their stock. Distemper did not disappear from London's dog population until Club Row market was finally shut down in the early 1980s. I'd visited the market during the previous summer and it was live theatre. I heard the yelps and yaps, the barks and howls well before I saw the dogs themselves. Up close the distressing whimpers hurt.

It wasn't just dogs in the market. There were men with cigarettes hanging from their mouths, their coat pockets full of kittens, row upon row of cages of songbirds and parrots, rabbits and guinea pigs. Litters of pups were displayed in children's cots or playpens, sometimes huddling quietly in straw-filled wicker or laundry baskets. There were adult sheepdogs, spaniels, greyhounds, terriers and bulldogs either straining on leads or sitting sullen-faced. I was told this is where stolen dogs got sold, although all traders at least in theory needed street-trader licences.

From the street-hawker's banter it was easy to believe that stolen dogs got sold here and hard to believe all the hawkers were licensed.

''Ello, mate. He's worth ten quid he is, but a fiver to you cos I want him to have a good home and you look like an educated gent. Got his pedigree here in me pocket.'

'These 'uns were born between the sheets, Sir. Real pedigrees, they are. Twenty quid. No? Make me an offer.'

'Don't have a girl, Sir? This little'un, she'll keep you warm at night.'

Most of the cloth-capped traders showed affection towards their stock. Maybe it was real, maybe not, but it was good for business.

After that summer visit, I hadn't returned. Club Row disheartened me. I didn't like seeing the dogs in particular, especially the adults, treated like farm livestock.

Now I was starting to wonder. Is Harrods any different? The only real difference is that Harrods shoppers are wealthier than Club Row shoppers.

After work I meet Rose in Leicester Square. I think its quirky that she wants to see whether it is still filled with rubbish from the dustmen's strike that was on when she left for Springfield in December. It still is.

'Can you imagine this ever happening at home?' she asks me, and I can't. Any municipality would just hire new garbage collectors.

We walk to the Criterion Theatre on Piccadilly Circus, followed by a choreographed mass of tens of thousands of swooping, chattering, pirouetting starlings.

'Now that's pure theatre,' I say, and Rose agrees, although she tells me that after seeing Alfred Hitchcock's *The Birds* when she was in high school she never again trusted more than two birds together.

'I've been here before,' I tell her as we enter the theatre.

'What did you see?' she asks.

'A cat. It had fleas.' She laughs and hits my shoulder. By now I had visited most theatres in the West End, all with cats employed for mouse control.

The play *Flint*, with Michael Hordern portraying a wayward Anglican vicar who is transformed by a simple Irish girl, also stars Vivien Merchant.

We have a late meal at the Soho Stockpot, the sister restaurant of the Chelsea Stockpot.

'You don't see acting like that back at home, not even New York,' I say, and Rose agrees.

'The Irish girl? At home, she'd be a star. Here? The depth of acting is so great I didn't even catch her name.'

Rose agrees with that too.

I hadn't the faintest idea that I would, two years later, marry 'the Irish girl'.

10

In February, I finally went to one of Johnson's dog-training classes at his 'clubhouse', the St John's Wood church hall, near Lord's Cricket Ground. Noel, the vicar, gave it to him to use each Monday evening. I wasn't impressed.

Is it because my family had no military tradition that I was raised as I was? I don't know. My school teachers certainly thought that punishment was a valid form of learning. I was strapped for minor misdemeanours, homework not brought in, throwing snowballs at girls, but neither of my parents ever raised a hand either in anger or retribution. They didn't use punishment with our dogs either. Sparky, Misty and Duchess, all Yorkshire terriers, were obedience trained using biscuits called Milkbones as rewards.

Obedience through punishment was how social order was maintained, so I was not surprised that Johnson, a recently discharged military police dog trainer, taught compulsion as the best way to train dogs. He wasn't cruel. I could see he enjoyed working with dogs, especially the large ones in his class. All wore choke chains. He taught 'Sit' by showing the owners how to push their dogs' rumps down. He showed people how to yank hard on the dog's lead to get its attention. 'Don't bribe your dog with rewards,' he admonished. 'You are the leader of the pack and your dog does what you tell him because he knows you mean business.' Instinctively I knew there must be other ways to train dogs. I was hoping to learn something new. I didn't.

I help animals start life. The dog lying at my feet right now, Plum, I helped to start life when her mother, my other dog Bean, needed a caesarean section to successfully give birth to her. Death is also part of what I do. I'd learned at Brian's that I can help dogs with a good death, a comfortable and timely one. But I also learned that I can be the cause of bad deaths. There is no more horrible a feeling than that. There was one death that, although it made me think I should give up veterinary medicine, also changed my mind about how we should treat wildlife.

Thursday was turnaround day at the surgery. Brian unloaded the dogs he had operated on the previous Wednesday. A couple of Labrador bitch spays were tethered in the surgery bookkeeper Gertrude's room awaiting an early pick-up by their owner. There was a young Poodle that had lost the blood supply to the top of her femur, the bone that attaches the hind leg to the hip bone. She had been in chronic pain, and Brian had sawn off the top of her femur to alleviate that pain. And there were two Yorkshire terriers. They had been recuperating from their surgery for two weeks. Both were born with twisted hind legs, 'tibial torsions' that led to them having slipping kneecaps, 'patellar luxations'. It meant they hopped rather than walked. Brian had developed a surgical technique in which he delicately cut out the prominent ridge on the tibia, the 'tibial tuberosity', made a groove on the front of the bone, where it should have been in the first place, and screwed the transplanted bone into its new home. When surgery worked, and it almost always did in Brian's hands, the dog regained normal use of the affected leg.

I still had to meet more surgeons before I realised that Brian's confidence, his coolness, his self-belief were typical of surgeons. 'If it's broken, I can fix it.' I was finding that I enjoyed more the detective work of medicine, that Arnold Levene gave me the name of every tumour I removed, that Jean Shanks gave me bacteriology results so I knew what was causing an infection or blood results that helped me narrow down why an animal was ill.

This was the day I first met Margaret, Duchess of Argyll, a woman who would continue to bring her pets to see me for the next twenty-two years.

'Be nice to her and she'll be nice to you,' Pat tells me as she hands me my appointment sheet at the start of consultations. 'Mr Singleton is seeing out the ops and there's never anything wrong with her dogs.' She leans towards me and whispers, 'I think that's an excuse.'

There were many elegant clients at Pont Street, but the Duchess arrived at 10 am looking as if she was going to a coronation. In her late fifties, my mother's age, so to me three paces short of deceased, she had lime green eyes and, from ear to ear, blown-back jet black hair swept four inches high like a rigid fur coronet. Around her neck were three strands of pearls and on her ears large, round pearl earrings. She wore a full-length black diamond mink coat and was followed into the consulting room by a chauffeur in grey cap, jacket and breeches, and black leather boots, carrying two black Poodles, whom I soon learned were Antoine and Pierre.

'Antoine and Pierre are not well,' she tells me, without a 'Hello' or any other introduction.

'Good morning. What are they doing to let you know they aren't well?'

'They refused to go out this morning,' she says, and I ask the chauffeur to put one of the dogs on the examination table.

'This is Antoine,' he tells me.

'Did they eat this morning?' I ask.

'Yes, they did. Is Mr Singleton too busy to see me?'

'I'm afraid he has a very sick dog and can't see anyone this morning,' I say and continue my physical examination of Antoine, who looks a happy, sparky individual. His temperature is normal.

'And body functions? Have they performed today?' I ask, and the Duchess tells me they both 'spent pennies' on the lamppost outside the surgery.

I examine Pierre, and he too looks, sounds and feels normal.

'It may be that they were feeling poorly this morning but perked up when you told them you were taking them to the vet.' Their owner's face remains mask-like, not the trace of a smile.

'They do hate rain, Your Grace,' her chauffeur adds. 'And it was quite dreadful earlier this morning.'

I am convinced there is nothing wrong with her dogs but feel I should do something. Frank's idea of a B12 injection for everything crosses my mind, but instead I say, 'They were obviously not well this morning, but fortunately are much better without my needing to do anything. I'm sorry Mr Singleton isn't free, but I'll discuss them with him and telephone you if he would like to see them back.'

At lunchtime I say to Pat, 'I didn't know they still make them like that,' and she says, 'Were you nice to her?' The dimples in her cheeks are cavernous, so I know she has something to tell me.

'You're getting at something,' I say.

'Well, in the past she's been known to service government ministers and Hollywood film stars, and give them Polaroids as souvenirs.'

'No. Really?'

'She's ostracised by society. And she's not the Duchess of Argyll, she's Margaret, Duchess of Argyll. She's the *former* Duchess. Her divorce was a juicy scandal, just before Profumo.'

'But she looks plastic.'

'Not in the 1930s. She was the most beautiful woman in Britain. Cole Porter wrote lyrics about her.'

'Wow,' is all I can say.

The only surgical case booked in is a road traffic accident I'd seen that Brian wanted to operate on, so I go upstairs to read the latest copy of the *Journal of the American Veterinary Medical Association* that has just arrived, but as soon as I sit down the intercom on the phone buzzes.

'The puma at Harrods is restless and drooling saliva. They'd like you to visit,' Jane tells me.

I fill my doctor's bag with cortisone, antibiotic and sedative injections, and run over to Harrods.

The cat has been there longer than Mr Grimwade expected. Now a mature cub, she is the size and weight of a female Border Collie and in a dire state, her head extended as far forward as she can get it, struggling with each inward breath. Her enclosure is surrounded by fabric screens on wheels.

'We need to get her to the surgery now,' I tell Grimwade.

'That will be difficult, Vet,' he says. 'We don't have a crush cage to get her in and we can't be seen taking her through the shop.'

'Phone the surgery and tell Pat to grab some thio* and a bunch of middle-size endotracheal tubes, and get over as fast as she can.'

'She's dying,' I tell him. 'She can't breathe,' and as I say that she stops breathing.

'Fuck!' I mutter. I am becoming British.

---

* 'Thio' or thiopentone is a fast-acting anaesthetic.

Her gums are blue. I listen to her heart. It is still beating. One habit I never lost was to carry a penknife in my pocket. I roll her onto her back, take out my penknife and cut through the hair on her neck over her windpipe. Nothing. The penknife doesn't penetrate her fur, let alone her skin. It's blunt.

Annabelle has been opening cardboard cartons. She runs over to them, runs back and hands me a Stanley knife. It cuts through the puma's skin in one slice, revealing her windpipe. I make an inch-long incision in her windpipe and hold it apart with the Stanley knife blade and my penknife. I tell Annabelle to press on her chest as if she is giving heart massage, but before she lays her hands on the cat's chest I hear a sucking sound. She breathes in on her own. She has a blockage in her throat or her larynx, but her lungs are fine. Soon colour returns to her gums and the puma blinks.

Now what? I think.

As if cued by an out-of-sight film director, the cavalry arrive at exactly the right time, but it isn't Pat with the endotracheal tubes, it's Brenda.

'Pat's helping Mr Singleton,' she explains.

Even better. Those kittens born without the parts of their brains they needed in order to balance themselves, the ones I helped suckle from their mother knowing what I was doing was in vain? Turns out it wasn't. Brenda had been right and I was wrong. By ten weeks of age, they were scampering around. Somehow, other parts of their brains had compensated for the missing parts. Brenda was my cat saviour.

'I got what you wanted and I've also got some of that anaesthetic we're testing. Mr Singleton told me to bring it. And Dexon. And a surgical kit, and a tracheostomy tube.'

CT1341 was a new injectable anaesthetic from Glaxo that we were doing clinical trials on. It was radically different from other general anaesthetics, a combination of two steroids, alphaxolone and alphadolone, which could be given intravenously but also intramuscularly. Glaxo called it Saffan when they eventually marketed it to vets.

The cat is now regaining consciousness, and I have only minutes before I can't control it.

'Brenda, draw up the anaesthetic. She's around twenty kilos, so 400 mg. Annabelle, put your hand around her elbow, fingers behind, thumb front, pull back and squeeze.'

As she does, I feel the vein in the cat's front leg go turgid with blood, and I slowly inject the anaesthetic until she is unconscious and breathing regularly.

Brenda hands me the silver-plate tracheostomy tube, opens the surgical pack and drops some Dexon on it. I sew the tracheostomy tube in place, reduce the size of the tracheal incision and then the skin incision.

'Mr Grimwade, I need a torch,' I say, and he returns with one. I look down the cat's throat. Its larynx is swollen tight shut. I prod it with the smallest endotracheal tube but can't get through.

'Something's caused an allergic reaction in her throat,' I say.

'I can't think what that might be,' Mr Grimwade replies.

'People give things to the animals. I see them,' Annabelle adds.

'Right,' I say. 'Immediate crisis over. Now we've got to get rid of that swelling in her larynx,' and I give the puma a corticosteroid injection and an ampicillin antibiotic injection.

'The tracheostomy tube should stay in for five to seven days. We'll need to give CT1341 to take it out, but that can be given intramuscularly.'

I arrange that I'd drop by after work, and Mr Grimwade tells me which door to go to so that I can be let in after hours.

There aren't many opportunities in veterinary medicine to immediately and instantly save a life. I did with Felicity's dog and now I'd done the same with the puma. Do I need to tell you how wonderful I feel? I bounce back to the surgery, skate through the afternoon appointments, visit the now back-on-her-feet, relaxed and comfortable puma after work, then race over to Rose's to tell her all about it.

I stayed at Rose's that night and am greeted by a red-eyed Brenda when I arrive at the surgery the next morning.

'It died.' She can't say more and leaves the room.

'They're sending the body over for a post-mortem,' Pat explains.

I am numb. It can't have happened? *What had I missed?*

Minutes later a Harrods van pulls up outside the surgery, and the driver and Annabelle carries in the puma, its rigid body, in rigor mortis, wrapped in a blanket.

'Downstairs, please,' I say, and take over from Annabelle, taking the cat down to the prep table.

'Annabelle, I'm so sorry.'

'We found her like this, this morning,' she says.

I unwrap the blanket, and her head is outstretched as it was when I first saw her.

'It's not right,' Annabelle says.

'No, it's not fair,' I reply.

'No, it's not right. We shouldn't keep beautiful wild things like this for our own amusement.' Her fingers are buried in the hair over the puma's shoulder. It is a throwaway line, Annabelle saying, 'It's not right.' She is talking to herself, not to me. But she is right. Harrods shouldn't be selling pumas or monkeys or alligators or skunks. People shouldn't keep wildlife as pets. It's wrong. Annabelle is right. I need her saying it to herself for me to actually think about it. And soon to do something about it.

'I'll do an autopsy at lunchtime and send a written report on why she died,' I tell her, and she returns to the driver and his van.

The morning's appointments passed in a blur. My mind kept flitting back to the puma. What had I missed? Why did she die so unexpectedly? Did she suffer?

Death seldom comes easily to animals. They rarely have strokes or heart attacks, the best deaths for us. They waste away, suffer nausea and start choking. The animal's body often holds on. Almost as soon as I started the post-mortem I knew why she died and that I was her killer. Cortisone had worked. The swelling in the larynx had dramatically reduced. Her lungs were perfect, just some spotty bleeding from the distress she had suffered. The only thing that was not right was the tracheostomy tube itself. It was plugged air tight with compacted glue-like mucus. If I had monitored her overnight, as I would have a dog, if I had regularly cleaned the tracheostomy tube with its own plunger, she would have lived.

I had left her to die alone and distressed. I had saved her, only to kill her twelve hours later.

11

For seven years I paid my annual tuition fees to study anatomy and physiology, and then pathology, how bad things can happen to the body. I was trained in the ever improving methods employed to stop those bad things happening, medically, by using drugs that had been developed to treat equivalent pathologies in humans, or surgically, by repairing or removing the pathology. As a student, I didn't think I needed to know more than that, just how to stop pathologies and make bodies better.

I've intentionally said that I had a veterinary *training*, not a veterinary *education*. I was trained in how to make logical and sensible diagnoses, how to intervene medically or surgically, but not to think about what I was doing. Surgery was like a bank heist. Smash and grab. An organ is irreversibly diseased? Remove it. A body part is damaged? Repair it. I was developing the technical skills to be a successful surgeon, but I loved the challenge of solving intricate problems, of creating in my mind a list of possible causes of a condition, then applying logic to single out which item in that list was most likely to be the vital one. I was learning for the first time that sometimes you have a problem and nothing on your list solves it. What happens when you can't solve an animal's health crisis? And what about ageing? We never discussed ageing. My education only started when I was confronted by the everyday realities of our sharing our lives with other animals. I learned that I had to confront natural ageing, inevitable physical decline and death. It was the nurses I worked with who made me think, who educated me.

Clem, a black Labrador, was born in May 1955. Clem's owner explains to me that he was named after Clement Attlee, the then leader of the Labour Party. 'Clem arrived on election day,' he says, 'just as his namesake departed from the prime minister's office. He was a quiet pup at first, no charisma whatsoever. Much like the original, but his faithfulness has been outstanding.'

Sixteen years old, Clem has been unable to stand up without assistance for several months. Now he can't stand at all and isn't eating. His owner carries him up the stairs and lays him on the examining table, where I can see that his muscles have wasted away and can smell an offensive odour on his breath. Clem's breathing is laboured and he has a vacant, distant look in his eyes. When I look in his mouth, I see that his teeth are covered in thick plaque, and his gums ulcerated and inflamed. I know that kidney failure is at least a part of his many problems. His kidneys are no longer ridding his body of toxic waste.

'I want you to do everything you can to save him,' his owner tells me. 'I can't bear the thought of losing him.'

'Right,' I answer. 'First I need to know exactly what medical problems he has. I can check his blood and urine, X-ray his chest to see why his breathing is laboured and keep him here for a few days on intravenous fluids to wash some of the toxins out of his blood stream. And I'll give him antibiotics and scale his teeth.'

'That sounds excellent. Do what you can. Don't worry about the costs. Just make him better.'

I ask the dog's owner to telephone the following day for the blood, urine and X-ray results, then carry Clem down to the kennels. At lunchtime I explain to Brenda and Pat what my plan of action is. They say nothing, to me or to each other, but continue with their separate tasks for a minute until Pat stops, turns and says, 'Bruce. What is Clem suffering from?'

I reply that he smells as if he has kidney failure, is dehydrated, has a bacterial infection to his gums and a lung problem I'll be able to identify once I X-ray his chest. 'His blood and urine results will tell me what else is going wrong,' I add.

'You're the vet, so it's your decision what needs to be done, but do you want my diagnosis of what Clem is suffering from?' Pat says. Brenda is quiet and intent. I nod my assent.

'Clem is not suffering from a grab bag of medical problems. You are turning a natural event into a differential diagnosis. Clem is simply old and he's dying of old age. You might want to break that down into infection and kidney failure and lung disease and muscle atrophy, but all you are doing is turning something normal into something medical. Not only that, but you plan to carry out tests and treatments he has no say in and that are, let's be honest, pointless.'

I say nothing, although I intuitively know she is exactly right. Then Brenda enters the conversation.

'Wendy, that old cat who just hated being here – hated it – who you kept on fluids all week just because her owner couldn't face her dying? I thought you were arrogant and callous. It was the natural end to her life. She must have felt as if we were virtually assaulting her every day, with the needless suffering she had to go through.'

Wendy's week of intravenous fluids had worried me too, although I didn't mention that to anyone. Brian had a firm ethical policy. We do diagnostics and treatments because the owners want them, never simply to bring added revenue into the surgery. But should I always do what owners want me to do? There's a constant conflict between what the owner wants, what's best for the animal, the vet's ego and the financial rewards of doing 'something'. We always hope that something can be done. We take from medical culture the hope that new treatments will work. Hope is within the very essence of who we are. But in some instances it is a foolish feeling.

'Okay,' I say. 'I agree with you. What do we do when someone wants something done and we know it's not in their pet's interest?'

'Argue on his behalf!' Brenda blurts. 'You're the vet. They'll respect you. Tell Clem's owner he's just being mean and selfish.'

'Bruce, you understand what Brenda is saying,' Pat adds. 'Guide Clem's owner towards what you think is the best option for Clem.'

I looked at Clem, lying in his kennel, breathing heavily, and felt embarrassed that I needed the nurses to tell me he was simply a smelly and enduringly loved, old dog who was now dying, and that I should help, not hinder. Pat telephoned Clem's owner, who returned and, with Pat and Brenda in the room to give me demonstrative support, I explained why it was not in Clem's interest for us to put him through what would be pointless diagnostics and treatments. 'It's better for him to end his life with dignity,' I conclude.

'May I take him home so his life ends in his own basket?' Clem's distressed owner asks.

'Of course.'

'And all of us will visit early this evening,' Pat adds. That was the only occasion when two nurses accompanied me on a visit.

12

A year in London and I was still making exciting new discoveries. The Roundhouse at Chalk Farm, where I saw Fairport Convention. Nearby Marine Ices on Chalk Farm Road, for amazing home-made ice cream. The fruit, vegetable and flower market in Covent Garden. Schmidt's restaurant on Charlotte Street for *gemütlichkeit*, cosy Middle European meals. Cranks on Marshall Street for organic food. The steam room in Seymour Baths on Seymour Place. The Sea Shell on Lisson Grove for fish and chips for twenty pence, where there was always a street dog hanging around for a little cod. Farringdon Road Book Market. The Brick Lane Beigel Bakery. I was loving life in central London. Brian's clients were the powerful and famous, but they didn't hold any allure for me. London itself was much more exciting.

'Crafty bugger. Do you fancy her?'

Pat always arrives before 8 am each weekday and is mopping the floor in the waiting room when I come down from my flat above the consulting rooms. On the nights I stay with Rose, I make sure I get back to the surgery well before any of the RANAs arrive.

Pat is grinning mischievously as I reach the bottom of the stairs. How does she know I am sleeping with a client?

'Who? What?' I say.

'Annabelle. Do you fancy her? She is quite pretty in a youth-ful, immature way.'

'What about Annabelle?' I say.

'Mr Singleton is hiring her. As if I didn't have enough to do training Brenda.'

'Hey, that's terrific!' I reply. 'She's great. Every time I go to Harrods she's done something that's impressed me. But why am I a crafty bugger?'

'Well, Brucie, I think you've kept going on and on about her because you fancy her.'

'If you're asking, do I fancy her as a girlfriend, the answer is "no", but if you're asking, do I think she can do something better than be a shop assistant at Harrods, the answer is "yes". I think our clients are in for a treat.'

'Well, whatever,' Pat says. 'With Jane gone, Annabelle starts work in two weeks and Mr Singleton wants Brenda to become a fully qualified RANA asap.'

'No problem there,' I say. 'She's already on her way to becom-ing you, another vet in disguise.'

Pat says nothing, but her dimples deepen as she breaks into a broad smile. In 1971, women vets were still rare. My school in Canada had just lifted its restriction of a maximum of three per class. In England and Scotland the number of women students was higher, but they were still in a tiny minority of students, let alone graduate vets. It would be another decade or more before women were present in sufficient numbers to shift my profession from a practical and utilitarian one to a caring and empathetic one. In the meantime, vets often learned their care and consideration for clients as well as patients from their RANAs. And Jane? She was an efficient nurse. I'm not sure she wanted to give up her job, but in a male-dominated profession pregnancy was a black mark. She had, in effect, been fired and Annabelle hired to replace her.

'I've had a look at the day book,' Pat continues. 'It's another "meet the stars" day for you, not that you'd notice.'

Pat's sarcasm was justified. Shortly after I started working for Brian I vaccinated a Dalmatian pup, and after the dog and owner left, the nurses crowded around asking, 'What was he like?' I said he was a pretty typical Dalmatian, exuberant, amusing – fun as I'd expect any healthy pup to be, but before I could continue Jane interjected, 'No, stupid! Paul! McCartney! Is it true? Have the Beatles really split up? Is he as nice as he seems to be?' It would be a few years before I was relaxed enough with my diagnoses to pay attention to the people who brought their pets to see me.

Pat crosses her arms and looks straight at me.

'Today, you're going to Wapping to give Elizabeth Taylor a manicure.'

'I'm what?'

'And Richard Burton a pedicure!' she pronounces triumphantly. He's filming *Under Milk Wood* but he's going to be there especially for you,' Pat continues.

Pat's ability to pull my leg is major league, but I have no idea what she is talking about. She sees the blank expression on my face and relents.

'Last year Mrs Grievson sold a Shih Tzu to Elizabeth Taylor – company for her other Shih Tzu and her Peke. My guess is she refused to come to Britain while her husband is filming here because of quarantine, especially now that it's a year. So Richard Burton – or someone he knows – found a loophole in quarantine restrictions. It seems that if their dogs remain on their boat, technically they haven't entered Britain so they don't have to go through quarantine. The dogs live on the boat moored at Wapping while he's filming in Wales.'

Pat looks intensely pleased with herself. 'Isn't it just wonderful what influence can buy? Mr Singleton has arranged that you, you lucky thing, visit the dogs on their boat at Wapping Pier twice a month, to check their health and cut their nails.'

'*I'm* to cut Elizabeth Taylor's dogs' nails?' I ask. 'You know when I cut little dogs' nails they always bleed.'

'Well, on this occasion, to show you how to do it, you can take a professional with you. I'll do the lunchtime ops with Mr Singleton and you can take Brenda.'

The morning's appointments are uneventful, and in dappled sunshine Brenda and I walked down to Sloane Square, took the District Line train to Whitechapel then changed to a Metropolitan Line train down to Wapping.

'This is where I grew up,' Brenda tells me on the Metropolitan train. She is both my guide and my proud medical bag carrier. We emerge from Wapping Station and walk a short distance along Wapping High Street to Wapping Pier, where an Edwardian motor launch over 150 feet long is moored in solitude.

'Bom dia!' a deckhand calls out as we walk down the narrow steel gantry to the boat's foredeck. The view from the deck is exactly why I am in no rush to leave London and return to Canada. Because of the bend in the river and the location of the boat's mooring, there is Tower Bridge, right in front of me, with trucks and cars slowly crossing as if they are driving right into the Tower of London.

Red, white, blue, yellow and black squared and triangular signal-flag bunting, fluttering in the crispy midday light, runs from the boat's bow up to a fore mast then an aft mast then down to the boat's stern. The boat itself is freshly painted brilliant white, with the words *Kalizma* and *Nassau* in black on the side of the bow and on large plaques above the wheel house. The raised anchor, also black, looks freshly painted.

'Ola. Veterinario?'

'Si. Vaca fala Ingles?' I ask.

Brenda leans over and whispers, 'What's he saying?' but before I can answer, the deckhand who asked if I was the veterinarian says, 'You're friend ask if cow speaks English.' We corpse with laughter. I figure I should retire the know it all, smart alec in me.

As we speak, two shaggy Shih Tzus, chewing each other's necks as they trot along, accompanied by a neater, smaller Pekingese, approach over the shellacked wooden deck and greet us with smiles and wagging tails. Brenda is the first to bend down to say hello, and they compete at her knees for her attention.

'Would you like to see the boat?' the 'deckhand' who is in fact the Portuguese captain asks, and each of us with a dog in hand is taken on a tour. I am most interested in the new Range Rover chained onto the top aft deck. I've seen photos of this just launched, new 4x4, but this is my first chance to see one up close. The captain is equally proud of it and opens the driver's door so I can look inside.

'All plastic and vinyl, you see. Is easy to hose down inside and out. Is Mr Burton's for going to Wales.'

On the lower aft deck are a variety of unmatched chairs but also warm sunshine, and that is where Brenda examines the dogs' nails and I examine their other parts. She shows me that the Peke's nails, the ones most in need of trimming, are translucent, so easy to cut without accidentally incising the living, bleeding quick. One of the Shih Tzus also has white nails, making accurate nail clipping easy, but the darker-coated dog has several dark nails. We use its white nails as guides to how much can be cut.

Brenda shows the captain how to hold the dogs firmly while she gives them their pedicures. She knows I'll need his help when I return next month. While she cuts their nails, I ask the captain why the boat is called *Kalizma*.

'Is for Miss Taylor's children, Kate, Liza and Maria,' he explains.

And somehow, that simple fact makes her instantly accessible. Surrounded by her dogs, naming her boat after her children, she is a mum, like mine but with more diamonds. My mother named our cottage on Lake Chemong *Braimoro*, after me, my parents Aileen and Morris, and my brother Robert.

'You come each week to cut nails?' the captain asks. 'They no good for deck.'

'Telephone us any time if there's a problem. I'll be back in two weeks to give them a check-up and cut their nails.' We shake hands, and Brenda and I return to shore.

'Do we have time for me to show you the best bit of Wapping?' Brenda asks. It will take a little over half an hour by train and foot to get back to the surgery, but that leaves us with almost forty-five minutes leeway. We turn right along Wapping High Street, then onto Wapping Wall and along an alleyway I would have missed if I had been there on my own, down towards the river to wooden stairs leading to the Thames. *Into* the Thames!

'I saw it was low tide and thought you'd find it funky to walk on the river bed,' Brenda explains. 'This is Pelican Stairs. Not many people use it, but this is where I went mudlarking when I was little. Still do. Love it.'

The river bed is solid, no mud, just pebbles and grit with dashes of red and mats of green vegetation.

'Walk out here and I'll show you why we come here,' Brenda says, and I follow her to the left, out to the edge of the receding tide then turn around and look back.

'That's the Prospect of Whitby pub. People have been losing things or throwing things into the Thames from there for hundreds of years. That's why you always find something interesting, no matter how often you visit.'

She bends down in a 'bunny dip', the only way to bend in a
RANA trainee uniform, surveys the river bed, and in less than
ten seconds picks up an object and shows it to me. It is the bowl
of a clay pipe.

'Clay pipes don't mean anything. Smokers threw them in the
river the way they throw cigarette butts today, but this is special
because its bowl is so small.'

'What's that mean?' I ask.

'It's really old, over a hundred years, from when tobacco was
really expensive.'

I bend down and survey the river bed, and as my eyes adjust
to looking at detail, I see it isn't just pebbles and grit. The wet
surface is also covered with broken red bricks and grey pottery,
and littered with parts of broken clay pipes.

'We always looked for dark mud,' Brenda continues. 'Digging
in dark mud is the most fun. I've sometimes found old buttons
or trader's tokens or coins in dark mud.'

My eyes scan the river bed. It reminds me of going to antique
shows while at college in Ontario, scanning the contents of
stalls, looking for the diamonds in the dross.

'Hey, look at this!' I shout. 'It's a whole clay pipe. And here's
a sixpence!'

'That's good,' Brenda says. 'They're your souvenirs for visiting my home.' I see pride in her eyes.

We ascend the stairs back to Wapping Wall, where Brenda
has one last location to point out to me before we take the tube
back to Pont Street.

'See that building across the street? That's Wapping Hydraulic
Power Station. Remember you told me it sounded like someone
had just flushed a toilet when we got in the lift at Cumberland
Mansions on Seymour Place when we visited those Siamese cats
last week?'

'Yes, I remember.'

'Well, that's because that lift is connected by pipes all the way here. This is where the flush is. When you pressed the "up" button in the lift, that flushed the machinery here to push the lift up. When you pushed the "down" button, it flushed again right here and the pipes emptied. If you ever go to a play in the West End, listen when the safety curtain goes up. They get flushed from here too.'

13

The British Small Animal Veterinary Association (BSAVA) held monthly lectures at the Royal Society of Medicine just north of Oxford Street. The lectures were always about veterinary techniques, never about the animals we were doing things to, never about how or why they behaved as they do. I didn't hear any talks about animal behaviour, or about the behaviour of the people who live with animals, until I organised a symposium on those topics for the BSAVA ten years later. Keith, Mike and John were usually at these evening meetings. I kept promising to visit their clinics, but because I worked the same hours they did, it was difficult. Brian was keen for me to suggest improvements at his surgery and he arranged that on Tuesdays, when I was on call for the rota all night, I could have an extended lunch break until 4 pm to visit other clinics. I was curious about Notting Hill. There had been race riots there the previous summer and John practised nearby, so I arranged to visit him at his surgery after morning appointments finished.

The morning went smoothly, but for a client whose dog urinated on her bed. I had seen the dog previously and treated her with antibiotics, but the problem continued, and now she was back with the urine sample I had asked for. I did a urine stick test and all was normal. No glucose, so the dog wasn't diabetic. Nicely concentrated, so the dog was secreting the hormone needed to concentrate urine. No unpleasant smell that might signal infection. No red or white blood cells or by-products of bacteria. Infection had been my first guess and the reason I had given the dog a new antibiotic, Septrin, that we were told was ideal for urinary tract infections. I didn't send the sample to Dr Shanks for culture and sensitivity because there was a continuing postal strike, now in its second month, and in 1971 the concept of a bike or motorbike courier service hadn't yet developed in London. I'd run out of medical reasons for what the dog was doing.

Brian had provided me with a record player in my flat upstairs, together with a small selection of LPs. All were classical music apart from one, which was instructional: *Dog Training My Way* by a woman named Barbara Woodhouse. The sleeve showed a handsome Great Dane sitting in front of a red brick stately home. On the back of the sleeve were black and white photos showing among other things the 'Correct way for choke chain' and 'Wrong way for choke chain'. Three pictures showed how to get a dog into a 'down' position. The first was captioned, 'Place left foot on lead on running end over choke chain.' The next instructed, 'Holding lead high in right hand exert pressure with left foot,' and the last one said, 'Keeping lead under arch of shoe release pressure when dog is down.' That was how dogs were trained then, with coercion. I didn't question these methods. Why should I? They seemed to work. If you discover that your puppy has peed in the house, push his nose in it and say, 'Bad dog!' If your dog pulls on its leash, use a choke collar or better still a prong collar so it hurts when he pulls. If he won't sit when you tell him to, push him down. At university, we never discussed animal behaviour. The subject wasn't 'scientific'. But now, in clinical practice, I was learning that virtually *all* pet owners had questions about their dog or cat's behaviour. All I could do was wing it, make it up as I went along, and my only sources were books by dog trainers like Barbara Woodhouse, or in this instance her record. I'd listened to the record but the instructions only covered 'Tone of voice' and 'Teaching your dog to ignore other dogs', not what to do when your dog peed on your bed. I could have told the client to push her dog's nose in the pee, but she told me she had already done this and it hadn't worked.

'Can you excuse me a moment?' I say to the dog's owner, and search out Brian, who was plastering the forelimb of a whippet that had been hit by a car. I explain what I'd ruled out.

'Any ideas?' I ask.

'Well, if it's a behaviour problem, that has nothing to do with us. Tell her to get in touch with Barbara Woodhouse. She runs two-day dog-training courses in Rickmansworth.'

That's what I did.

After morning appointments I walked down to Sloane Square, took the Circle Line train to Notting Hill Gate and walked down Holland Park to John's surgery on Addison Avenue. If local property had been damaged during the previous summer's race riots, it had all been repaired. Holland Park looked as affluent as Belgravia.

John's surgery is even smaller than Brian's, a tiny four-seat waiting room and office at the shop's front, with a single consulting room behind. Down a steep and tight staircase there is, to the right, a narrow room lined with wooden kennels and, to the left, an operating room with a coal cellar beyond. John is already operating when I enter the room.

As I am about to say 'Hello', his RANA puts her finger to her lips, silently instructing me to remain silent. The cat John is operating on has an ether mask on her face and is on her side, covered in a green laparotomy cloth. I can see that John has made his skin incision and withdrawn one horn of the uterus. His hands are poised over the surgical site but they are not moving. He is as still as a statue. I look over to his RANA and again she puts a finger to her lips. John remains frozen, then gradually his hands start to move and he deftly continues operating.

'Bruce, hello. This is my last op. I'll be finished shortly and we can have lunch.'

John finishes the spay. His surgery is neat and tidy.

'Good. Let's go upstairs and chat. Would you like some yoghurt? I make my own.' Yoghurt is still an exotic food in Britain in those days, something to discover when visiting Greece.

We walk over to a bird incubator John has in the corner of his operating room, he takes a cloth-covered bowl from it and then, taking three steps at a time, flies upstairs. I turn to his RANA behind me. 'He meditates,' she says.

I already knew I wasn't going to provide Brian with new ideas gleaned from John's surgery, but over a lunch of bird-incubator yoghurt, cereal grains and dried fruit in his flat upstairs, we talk shop. I tell John about the dog that peed on the bed and he suggests that the behaviour might be caused by a dietary deficiency. 'Are they feeding the dog commercial food?' he asks, and I don't have an answer because diet was a question I asked about only when a dog or cat had a gastrointestinal problem. It would be some years before vets learned that diet is a common aggravating factor in many conditions, particularly itchy-skin problems.

'You might want to try this,' John says, and he gets up from the kitchen table and takes a small brown paper bag from a cupboard filled with identical bags.

'What is it?' I ask.

'Comfrey root. Last summer's. I grow it out the back.'

I open the bag and see it contains dried, coarse vegetable matter.

'How does it work?'

'It calms the bladder. It's particularly useful for cats with cystitis. It may work on your dog.'

It didn't, but after John retired young to Scotland and opened a herbal veterinary practice in which he consulted by telephone with clients in London, I referred many owners to him of cats with bladder irritation, and they were invariably satisfied with the results of his dried-herb treatments.

That evening Rose came to the surgery and made dinner. Juicy, thick hamburgers, followed by pastry from Harrods for dessert. We talked about nothing in particular, but I could see she was pensive, more restrained than I had seen her. After we finished our meal, she came over, sat on my lap and put her arms around my neck.

'I think I might be going home,' she says.

'Why?' I ask. 'You were just home a few months ago.'

'My mom. Something's happened and she's not right. My dad thinks seeing me will help.'

'Stay the night.'

'No. Bobby is on his own,' she replies.

We washed and dried the dishes together, and she left.

Late the following morning, Mick Bullock trots in and places a large brown bag containing three kittens on the receptionist's desk. 'Found 'em in the rubbish in Eaton Square.' Mick is our local dustman on Pont Street. When I set up my own clinic in 1973, near Marble Arch on the north side of the Royal Parks, Mick followed me there. It suited him as he lived on the Lisson Green Estate, ten minutes north of Marble Arch.

Brenda is on reception and brings the kittens and Mick up to me. The kittens look around three weeks old.

'You found these in Eaton Square?' I ask.

'That's right, mate. Someone tossed 'em out,' Mick says.

'Are you sure they didn't stray from their mother?'

'Into a dustbin with its lid on?' Mick asks.

All three, all females, looked well fed and healthy.

'The poor mother,' Brenda says. 'She must be fretting over what's happened to her babies.'

'Do you think we can find her?' I ask.

'Already tried, Vet,' Mick injects. 'Me and me mates, we knocked on all the doors. No one owned up to it. Cute little things, they are,' and with his stubby, blackened forefinger he rubs the head of the black and white kitten I have in my hands.

'Listen, mate, if they're healthy, me and me missus will have 'em. That's all I brought 'em here for. To see if they're healthy.'

'Brenda, they still need hand feeding. What do you think?' I ask.

'They do,' she answers, then turns to Mick. 'I can take them home until they're ready to go to your home.'

'Don't you have enough already?' I ask. 'And besides, they look healthy but they may be incubating infection. Maybe we should keep them here.'

'I don't think so,' Brenda says. 'If they're incubating infection, you don't want them in the kennels.'

All of us stare silently at the kittens for a moment, then Brenda says, 'Miss Williams. I'll ring Miss Williams and see if she can have them.'

'Who's Miss Williams?' I ask.

'She's a cat lady. In Mayfair.'

Veterinary medicine has changed dramatically from the time I worked for Brian, but 'cat ladies', usually but not always women, who collect cats in their homes, feed stray cats, invest in the welfare of cats, live and breathe cats sometimes to the detriment of their own physical or financial health, remain part of life at many vet clinics.

Brenda telephoned Miss Williams, discovered that by sheer good luck she only had her three resident cats in her home and arranged to take the kittens over after work. Miss Williams will hand feed them until they are old enough to move in with Mick and his wife. I asked Brenda if I could come along, so at 6.30 that evening, with our 'brollies', as I now called them, unfurled to protect us from the drizzle, we took the number 137 bus up Park Lane onto Oxford Street, getting off with our bundle of kittens at Selfridges.

'How do you know Miss Williams?' I ask Brenda on the bus, and she tells me that Miss Williams captures feral cats and brings them to Mr Singleton to be spayed or castrated.

'I don't know why he does it,' Brenda continues. 'He hates wild cats, and I have to shove them up the sleeve of a lab coat for him to get the ether mask on them. She keeps bringing more in because he never charges her. The only reason you haven't met her is because she's been ill for almost a year. She's better now.'

'We should use CT1341 on the next ones,' I suggest. 'It can be given intramuscular.'

It is dark when we arrive. Brenda has visited before and knows which of the many ill-lit entrances to the grimy red-brick block lead to Miss Williams's raised ground floor flat.

'Hello, hello, hello. Come in, come in,' Miss Williams cheeps when she answers the door. Inside there is a pervasive odour of tom-cat urine, although all of Miss Williams's resident cats had been castrated. She is a tiny woman with unorganised greying hair and lips like dried figs.

'Thank you, thank you,' she says, as Brenda gives her the blanket-covered wicker cat carrier containing the kittens. She draws back the blanket to see the kits.

'Beautiful, beautiful. Black and white. Beautiful.'

She lifts and inspects each one, giving particular attention to their bottoms.

'All females. Three weeks old. Good. Good.'

'We have a home for all of them once they're ready to go,' Brenda tells her.

'Good. Good. Five weeks,' she replies.

'What will you feed them with?' I ask, and when Miss Williams turns to me I see, disconcertingly, that one of her eyes is brown and the other hazel. I'd only ever seen that in a calico cat.

'Goat's milk and oatmeal. Then coley. Oh, hello there.'

'Hello, Miss Williams. I'm Bruce Fogle, a vet at Mr Singleton's.'

'Hello. How do you do?' she replies, offering me her hand. 'Would you like tea? Biscuits?'

'Thanks, but I'm meeting my girlfriend shortly. We're very grateful that you can look after these kittens. Do you have feeders you can use?'

She takes me through a lounge filled with books and porcelain figures and into her kitchen.

'I use these,' she explains, showing me a selection of fountain pen ink-fillers. 'I got this at Selfridges,' showing me a doll's feeding bottle, 'but it doesn't work as well.'

'Wow. That's very inventive,' I say. 'A company is producing rubber teats and small glass bottles for hand-feeding pups. We've got some at the surgery if you want to have a look.'

'Yes. Yes. I will,' she says.

'Brenda, are you happy with everything?' I ask.

Brenda is, so we thank Miss Williams for her help, and arrange that Mick and his wife come in a month and pick up their new kittens.

On Balderton Street, Brenda turns to me and says, 'She likes you.'

'How do you know?' I ask.

'She noticed you. Usually she doesn't notice anything but cats.'

14

Dog shows. From the very first one I saw in London, I didn't like them. It wasn't that the dogs being shown were mistreated. It was obvious that many enjoyed the sociability of dog shows. They were, just, well, icky.

'Bruce, Hilda and I are visiting Stockholm next week,' Brian tells me. 'We have a senior Cambridge student attending the surgery, so he will be your responsibility.'

'When does the student arrive?' I ask.

'Tomorrow.'

'You've given me tomorrow afternoon off to go to Crufts Dog Show. Does he stay here with you or go with me?'

'Take him with you. It will give you both the opportunity to develop your own impressions of dog shows. You should see Jane Grievson there, and if you see Mrs Wax, perhaps she might like to know you have intentionally visited to see her dogs.'

Meredith Lloyd-Evans arrived the next day just after I had started the morning consults. He had glossy and straight brown hair that flowed down onto his shoulders, a moustache straight out of *Viva Zapata!* and round, horn-rimmed glasses as thick as the bottom of a Coke bottle. His form-fitting, cream satin shirt had rounded collars. I am now wearing slightly flared trousers, but his are so flared they'd buoy him up if he fell in the Thames.

We had senior students visit the surgery regularly, an educational requirement called a 'preceptorship' that had to be completed before graduation. All the students I'd met were variations on the same theme: bright, conservative, middle class, middle of the road, in their early twenties but already middle-aged men. Meredith wasn't one of them. We briefly introduced ourselves to each other, then I continued with appointments.

'Which strain of distemper virus is in that vaccine?' Meredith asks after I give a booster inoculation to one dog.

'It's the Onderstepoort strain,' I answer.

'From Hoechst?' he asks.

'Yes.'

'From what I've read, their vaccine provokes high antigenicity. How long do you think it gives protection for?'

'Hoechst says a year.'

'Well, they would, wouldn't they, as Mandy Rice-Davies would say. What do you think?'

'I haven't thought about it,' I say. 'What do you think?'

'Well, logically,' he says, 'it must give protection for much more than a year. I wouldn't be surprised if, as long as a dog is injected after all maternally derived antibodies are gone, it gives lifelong protection.'

He's a bigger know-it-all than I am.

After a cat owner to whom I had dispensed an aerosol flea spray leaves, Meredith asks me why I have done so.

'It'll be warm soon. The BSAVA recommends routine parasite control,' I tell him.

'The owner mentioned now that she's opening her windows, she worries that her cat might fall out, so that cat never goes outside,' he comments.

'Well, there's no harm,' I say.

'It's an acetylcholinesterase inhibitor. The Soviets stockpile it as a nerve gas,' Meredith says.

'Does that mean fleas grab their throats because they can't breathe, have explosive diarrhoea, then cramp up and drop dead? I ask.

'If it does that to fleas, I'm just wondering what else it does to cats, other than kill fleas,' Meredith replies.

After all the appointments finished, we went across the road to Express Dairy and got ourselves cold Cornish pasties. Taking a bite out of his, Meredith says, 'In Wales this is sometimes called an *oggy*, from the Cornish *hogen*.' We munch lunch while walking down Sloane Street to Sloane Square, and take the District Line train, changing at Earl's Court for the special train to Olympia.

Malcolm Hime had told me he would meet me in the veterinary surgeon's room at 1.30 pm. Malcolm is an 'Honorary Veterinary Surgeon' at Crufts, there to inspect all dogs before they are shown, or so I assumed. The room was tiny, and after I met Malcolm and introduced Meredith to him, I asked where dogs are examined.

'We are not here to examine dogs,' he explains. 'We are here to treat bite wounds or collapsed individuals. Both are rare.' He continues, 'I have a suggestion for you. Barbara Woodhouse has a stand here. Perhaps you can ask her why the wolf peed on your trousers when I asked you to obtain that blood sample from him.'

I could see from the look in his eyes that Malcolm still enjoyed that joke on me. It had been a simple lesson on my second day at the zoo. A wolf had been brought the evening before to a large walk-in holding kennel at the zoo hospital and, almost as soon as I arrived for my first proper day of work, handing me an elastic limb tourniquet, Malcolm told me to collect a blood sample from it. I thought that would be dangerous, but nevertheless I walked down the hospital corridor to the holding kennel where the dog wolf was restlessly pacing back and forth. He kept his eyes on me as I slid back the two bolts on the door, entered the kennel and shut the door. He kept pacing, then suddenly lunged towards me, rearing up and placing his forepaws on my shoulders. It was frightening, but when I checked to see why my trousers were warm and wet, it wasn't me. The wolf had peed on me. I unbolted the door and escaped into the corridor, where Malcolm was waiting.

'If I hadn't asked you to do so, would you have ever entered a wolf's den?' he asks, and sheepishly I say, 'No.'

'Here at the zoo, all of us must always use our common sense. Think before you do anything.' He knew that the wolf was a hand-reared and very subservient youngster who loved human companionship.

'Come. I'll introduce you to some of the officers of the Kennel Club,' he says, and we follow him across the corridor to a larger room where a slice of middle England is eating sausage rolls and drinking sherry.

'John, this is Mr Fogle. He is Brian Singleton's assistant. And Mr Lloyd-Evans, a senior student at Cambridge.'

Malcolm turns to us. 'Mr Hodgman is Director of the Canine Health Centre at the Animal Health Trust.'

Staring straight into my eyes, John Hodgman grabs my hand and gives it a powerful shake.

'Good afternoon. You must have exceptional abilities if Singleton has selected you. Brilliant man. I'm still trying to convince him to leave his Knightsbridge ladies and join us. And good day to you too, Sir.' He turns to Meredith and shakes his hand.

'I very much enjoyed your article on abnormalities and defects in pedigree dogs,' Meredith comments.

Brown-nose!

'You shall certainly see some of those here,' he replies with a wide grin and a deep laugh.

'Mr Hodgman was a colonel in the Indian Army,' Malcolm tells us as we sip our sherries. 'Mr Woodrow was the first President of the BSAVA, Mr Singleton was the third and Mr Hodgman was the filling in between them.'

'Ah, our Chairman,' Malcolm says, seeing another familiar face. 'Founded the Alsatian League of Great Britain.' He walks us over to an erect man in a blue pinstripe suit, someone I judge to be the same age as my oldest uncles.

'Commodore, may I introduce Mr Fogle, Brian Singleton's assistant, and Mr Lloyd-Evans, a senior student at Cambridge. Air Commodore Cecil-Wright is Chairman of the Kennel Club.'

We shake hands.

'The Commodore served in the Royal Flying Corps in World War I and has been a Conservative Member of Parliament,' Malcolm tells us.

'Good afternoon, Sir,' I say. 'One of my uncles also served in the Royal Flying Corps in World War I.'

'His name?' the Chairman asks.

'Fogle. Myer Fogle. He volunteered for the Canadian Expeditionary Force and trained at Camp Borden, north of Toronto.'

'Odd Christian name. Don't think I ever met the man. Let me introduce you to one of my committee,' and the Chairman turns to another pinstripe-suited man he has been conversing with.

'Richard, this is Mr Fogle, Brian Singleton's assistant. Mr Fogle, meet Colonel Sir Richard Glyn. Sir Richard resigned his seat in parliament last year. Conservative, of course. Bull terriers.'

We shake hands.

'And this is Lloyd-Evans. He's completing his veterinary studies at Cambridge.'

There is more hand shaking.

'Which college are you at?' Meredith is asked.

'Churchill College,' he says.

'Is it new? I don't know it,' Sir Richard says, but before he gets an answer he turns towards another man who has just entered the room.

'Beefy! I was told you couldn't be here!'

Beefy, smiling broadly, joins us.

'Beefy, this is Fogle. He's Brian Singleton's assistant. And Lloyd-Evans, a senior veterinary student at Churchill College, Cambridge. Group Captain Sutton. He's a small terrier man,' Sir Richard explains.

A short, stocky man, another establishment Englishman, as Christopher Grievson would describe him, in matching pinstripe suit joins us. I am standing in a cartoon of Colonel Blimp's Britain! An Ealing comedy, but this one's for real.

'Sir Dudley,' Malcolm intones. 'Are you enjoying the show?'

'Good day, gentlemen. Very much so,' he replies, and he too is introduced to Meredith and me.

Meredith enjoys this banter and enthusiastically joins in. Whatever they are talking about, he has a lucid comment to add. I feel out of place. Eventually, I catch Meredith's eye and we tactfully excuse ourselves to return to the dog-filled halls.

'Do you know Sir Dudley Forwood's back history?' Meredith asks me later.

'He was the Duke of Windsor's equerry after his abdication in 1937,' he informs me. 'He may look like Colonel Blimp, but in his time he was a handsome man. He met the Duke and Wallis Simpson while skiing in Kitzbühel.'

I glare at him. 'Meredith, how do you know all this stuff?'

'Well, it's just general knowledge. The ruling classes are the members of the Kennel Club and those showing dogs are the oiks. It's harmless. And amusing, don't you think?'

We decide to head for the Utility Dog section. My programme tells me where Mrs Wax's dogs would be, but first we walk the aisles of exhibitors. We inspect a multi-vitamin supplement called Tonavet from Bimeda Chemicals. '*A Tonavet dog is fortified against nervousness and has greater resistance in times of sickness*,' the sign claims.

'Have they scientifically proven that?' Meredith asks.

Crest, a pure seaweed from Sea Products Research Ltd in Bristol, '*assists skin and coat condition, pigmentation and improves bone structure*'. Ashley's Gay Dog Coats has bargains in sub-standards. Dansie from Glasgow is selling silver car mascots in the breed of your choice. At another stand, an aluminium dog guard for your car costs £8, but one for a more pedestrian Austin Maxi is only £4. Joyce Cowen paints your dog's portrait on your scarf or your tie. Feeding your dog Wuffitmix will cost you six pence a day if you own a Poodle or one shilling and five pence if you feed an Alsatian. Shaw's Veterinary Chemists sell Everfree as a '*combined conditioner and worm preventative*'. Kanox Dog Foods promotes its Pure Full Cream Milk for bitches and Kanox Milk Equivalent for pups. 'What does "equivalent" mean?' Meredith asks on scanning the label, but there is no written answer and we don't stop and ask.

This man asks as many questions as my closest cousins.

Dog foods called Husky, Jessie, Luda and Dinnadog are for sale. So are Krunchy Dog Sticks, '*By appointment to Her Majesty Queen Elizabeth*'.

Pelham Books have a stand selling their dog-owner guides, encyclopaedias and Frank Manolson's books. I have no idea that ten years later I'll be visiting Jenny Derham at her Pelham editor's office in Bedford Square, discussing my own series of books for her. Nor when Meredith and I stop at the National Canine Defence League stand that in two years I will become their neighbour on Seymour Street, just north of Marble Arch.

Having been told about Barbara Woodhouse by both Malcolm and me, Meredith is interested in meeting her. Studying our Crufts programme, he knows where she is and sees her stand before I do.

'Mrs Woodhouse, I'm a senior veterinary student and this is Bruce Fogle, a vet who refers dogs to you for your excellent training course,' he interjects during a lull while she is speaking to a horseshoe of attentive women. 'He has a question for you about dogs that pee on their owner's beds.'

She smiles at Meredith and continues to speak to her congregants, but once she has finished – the point she was making was that dogs must know you are leader of the pack – she turns to us.

Barbara Woodhouse is a brunette, soon to be all grey, with neck-length, naturally curly and thick hair severely parted on the left. Ten years later, when she becomes a national celebrity through her TV series *Training Dogs the Woodhouse Way*, she is a parody of the asexual, no-nonsense, tweed-skirted, sensibly sweatered English governess, but on her stand at Crufts she oozes vitality.

'Where do you vet?' she asks, and I explain I am Brian Singleton's assistant.

'Fine man,' she replies. It seems that mentioning Brian's name at Crufts is like having a *Get Out of Jail Free* card.

'If you send the dog to me, I will train it to pee outdoors. Has it been fixed?'

'I can't actually remember,' I say.

'Fix it, then send it to me,' she replies, and, smiling, she turns to others waiting to speak to her.

The Miniature Poodles are in the next hall. We walk into it, getting our bearings on which aisle to head towards from the bench number cards provided by Chum, the dog food sponsor of Crufts. I point out Mrs Wax as we approach, and she is not the only perfectly coiffed Poodle breeder. Most of the women sitting at their benches are as neatly trimmed as their dogs.

'Mitzi!' I exclaim when I see her. 'What a nice surprise to see you here. Hello, Mrs Wax. This is Meredith Lloyd-Evans, a student doing practice with us.'

'Good afternoon, Mrs Wax,' Meredith adds. 'I must say, you look as delightful as your dogs do.' Mrs Wax beams at Meredith, who oozes charm like the slithery Hungarian count in *My Fair Lady*.

'I didn't know Mitzi was competing,' I say.

'She qualifies as a post-graduate, but I've entered her not for competition. She simply adores being here.'

I didn't understand what 'not for competition' meant but didn't ask for an explanation.

'How's everything gone?' I ask.

'Hattie did well but not well enough to reach best of breed,' she says. 'Mind you, the bitch the judge preferred is nothing to write home about. She'll be blind by the time she's Mitzi's age.

'Why is that Mrs Wax?' Meredith asks.

'Cataracts,' Mrs Wax smiles. 'Her mother will have cataracts. Mr Startup told me.'

This isn't unusual. In the 1970s around 10 per cent of all miniature and toy Poodles I saw developed cataracts while quite young.* Large numbers of both breeds were also blinded at a relatively early age, certainly before they were eight years old, by a hereditary condition called progressive retinal atrophy or PRA.

'And how's Trixie doing?' I ask. I'd done a pregnancy check and knew she was due to whelp in not much more than ten days.

---

* It wasn't until the Kennel Club, together with the BVA, offered specialist eye exams to certify breeding stock to be clear of this inherited problem that it disappeared.

'She's at home with Mr Wax,' Mrs Wax says.

Eventually we say our goodbyes and return to the commercial exhibition.

'Doesn't it seem odd to you,' Meredith asks as we walk the aisles, 'that a mother's milk does not contain enough calcium for the healthy development of her pups?'*

'I've never thought about that,' I say. 'But yes, there's no logic to it.'

'Everyone supplements their pups with sterilised bone flour, or products like Vivomin. I wonder whether it's really necessary?'

'I wouldn't think so for small pups like toy Poodles, but the giant breeds, they're man-made creations. Nature wouldn't grow dogs as fast as those pups grow. They probably need a calcium supplement,' I say.

'But nature grows other young even faster,' Meredith continues. 'If a foal gets all the nourishment it needs from its mare, why can't a Great Dane pup get all it needs from its mother?'

'Why isn't Mr Singleton here?' Meredith asks as we browse books on the Doggie Hubbard's Bookshop stand. 'It's obvious that he's a star of the dog world.'

'We can ask him tomorrow,' I tell him.

The following morning when Brian arrives for work, he asks Meredith and me to join him in his consulting room.

'What was your impression of Crufts?' he asks us.

'It's a curious mix,' Meredith answers before I can say anything. 'On the one hand, it appears to be the hobby of the retired great and the good, the self-satisfied and the verbose. And on the other hand, it produces enjoyment for breeders and their dogs.'

---

* The bit of trivia here is that it wasn't until the next year, 1972, when a Swedish vet Ake Hedhammar published his PhD thesis, that the idea of calcium supplementation started to die away.

'Did you come to any conclusions about the dogs that are shown at Crufts?' Brian asks.

'I was a bit surprised that there were no health checks,' I reply. 'The Honorary Vets there treated it more like a social event than anything else.'

'Mr Singleton, now that you mention it, your client Mrs Wax told us that the best in her breed would probably develop cataracts,' says Meredith. 'It's a shame that a dog that is seen as the epitome of its breed might carry such a devastating inherited condition.'

'Brian, does that have anything to do with your not being there?' I ask.

His answer is tactful. 'The veterinary members of the Kennel Club understand the problem, but they have a battle that will take at least a generation before the Kennel Club promotes good health as much as good looks.'

'Why so long?' I ask.

'The Kennel Club is quite military in its management,' he replies. 'The Show Committee are the officers and the breeders are their cannon fodder. Virtually none of the breeders you saw yesterday are members of the Kennel Club. If you visit a Swedish Kennel Club show, not only are all the exhibitors members of their kennel club, virtually every single Swedish dog owner is a member. And dog owners want good health as well as good looks. Their breeding dogs are examined for cataracts and PRA, and have their hips X-rayed for hip dysplasia if those are problems in their breeds. We are probably a decade away from doing so here.'

15

Few of us have the presence of mind to realise when a series of what are outwardly unrelated and pretty banal events are in fact life-changers. It was years before I realised that the week after Meredith (or Mery, as I would come to call him) left was one of the most important in my life. I learned more, in a concentrated period, than I would ever do again. Of course, I was still at the outset of my life as a grown-up and also as a vet. Empty containers are easy to fill. But during that week I had practical experiences that crystallised many of the thoughts and ideas I still hold today. And I met someone who would force me to confront who I was and where my future would be.

Monday started miserably. A dog had electrocuted itself on a live rail in Victoria Station. When a British Rail driver brought the body in I recognised Tweed, a young lurcher belonging to an actress client who lived just off the Kings Road. In my youth growing up in Toronto, my parents had allowed Angus, our Scottie, to roam freely all day but would never think of doing so with our Yorkshire terriers. That wasn't just because if the city dog-catcher caught them the fine was considerable. It was because our dogs had somehow ingratiated themselves into our lives. We allowed them on the furniture. When I came home from university, Misty, the meekest, slept on my bed – under the covers. Shouldn't all of us be more responsible about our dogs?

Later that morning, I am interrupted during a simple but wrought consultation with a bruiser of a man, a professional wrestler, and his overweight Bulldog, in for its annual distemper jab. After I examine Cassius, I get a vial of vaccine from the fridge, a disposable needle and syringe that we now used, and draw the vaccine out of the vial into the syringe. As I do so, I hear and feel the floor shake, turn around and find the wrestler out cold. He has fainted at the sight of the needle.

I go out into the hallway. 'Pat!' I shout, and Pat comes up the stairs, instantly assesses what has happened and turns Cassius's owner onto his side into the recovery position. Cassius casually sniffs his prostrate owner, and Pat looks up at me and grins. 'You're here to help, not frighten them to death.'

As the hulk starts to regain consciousness, Annabelle rushes in. 'There's an Alsatian with its foot stuck in the escalator at Knightsbridge Station!'

'Bruce, I'll look after Mr Breakspear. Take thio, 20 ml syringes, 21-gauge needles, alcohol, a large endotracheal tube, tape and gauze. If there's a taxi take one, otherwise do a fast walk. Annabelle, you go with him to raise the vein. The Fire Brigade will be there. Have them bring you back here and tell them to use their claxon so we know you're arriving. Mr Singleton will see your appointments, then when you get back you'll see his. He'll do the surgery. He likes escalator injuries.'

It is a drizzly day and there are no available taxis, but it takes less than five minutes to whizz up Sloane Street to Knightsbridge Station, where a crowd of Underground staff, firemen and passengers surround the top of the escalator. The dog, a young male well over forty kilogrammes, is sad and silent, being comforted by his owner who has his arm wrapped around the dog's chest.

'He knows he's supposed to lift his feet when he gets to the top, but this time he didn't,' the owner explains.

Arsehole, I think, then smile to myself. A little more of England's unpretentious vulgarity is seeping into me.

The dog's foot is impaled through the pad. In its struggle to get free, the dog has torn skin and tendons.

'Sir, once you've anaesthetised the dog we'll dismantle the equipment,' the nearest fireman says.

'Annabelle, go around to the other side of the dog so that both of you are holding him tightly and wrap your arm under his neck to lift his head up. Because his foot is caught, I'll be able to raise the vein and give the anaesthetic in that leg.'

Annabelle asks the owner the dog's name.

'Genghis,' he answers.

'Hello, Genghis,' she says to the dog in a soft, soothing voice. 'Poor Genghis. It's not your fault, Genghis. We'll get you sorted in no time, Genghis.' Annabelle intuitively understands how important it is that Genghis isn't frightened by her. She holds him firmly to her chest.

I swab the leg to flatten the hair and make his vein visible, and slowly inject the barbiturate anaesthetic. Without any premedication, the dog goes through an animated stage of excitement just before he falls asleep, going rigid, struggling and crying out. That upsets people watching, including Annabelle, and I explain to her that an excitement stage is normal.

'It'll be heavy, but now lift up his head with your fingers under his top jaw,' I tell Annabelle, and she does so in a resolute and convincing way. I pull out Genghis's tongue and ask Annabelle to hold it out with her other hand. Then, feeling his larynx through the skin on his neck, I blindly guide the endotracheal tube into his windpipe and inflate it.

'Great, now let's get a syringe in his good leg,' I tell her, and we place a fresh syringe with fast-acting thiopentone in the other leg and tape the syringe securely in place.

'Okay. He's yours,' I tell the firemen, and with bolt removers, a massive screwdriver and sledgehammers it takes them less than five minutes to dismantle the grate at the top of the escalator and free Genghis's foot. There is surprisingly little bleeding. I wrap the foot in bandage, as much to keep the ticket hall at the tube station tidy as to control bleeding, and with the help of a fireman carry Genghis to the fire truck outside the station, where they suggest that we lie him on the front seat beside the driver. I get in and kneel with him while Annabelle and the dog's owner walk in the continuing drizzle back to the surgery.

'Fucking arsehole,' the driver says as he does a U-turn. I feel great. The driver's on my team. With claxon sounding we head down Sloane Street. 'While you're at it, why don't you remove the fucking git's bollocks. Dog like that on an escalator. Can you save his foot?'

'I'm sure we'll save every toe,' I say. 'The best surgeon in the country is waiting for him.'

Mr Breakspear, the needle-phobic wrestler, had revived and departed by the time we arrived back at the surgery. The waiting room was full of pet owners and pets, as Brian had been seeing both his clients and mine. Genghis started to recover from his initial anaesthetic on the short drive to the surgery and I had given him more thiopentone through the strapped-on syringe. With the fireman's help, we carry him downstairs and place him on the operating table, where I hook him up to our pristine halothane vaporiser. Brian joins us, examines the damage and I see him wince when he counts the number of torn tendons.

'Thank you, Bruce. Well done. This will take some time, but I expect a good outcome.' I go up to the waiting room and explain this to Genghis's now very sheepish-looking owner.

'The firemen told him what they thought you should do to him,' Pat whispers to me in the hallway, her dimples deep with satisfaction, knowing that although we might have to be diplomatic, they don't.

I leapt up the stairs to my consulting room, then worked through the backlog of waiting pets and their people. Most were simple visits, routine annual health checks, itchy skin or booster inoculations, but one case worried me a little. I had noticed the Golden Retriever in the waiting room when we carried the anaesthetised German Shepherd through it on our way downstairs to the operating room. The dog's owner, a small woman, not much more than my mother's height, five foot two inches, my age, with an awful lot of cascading blonde hair, is not happy to see me.

'Why can't I see Mr Singleton?' she asks.

'I'm sorry but he has an emergency operation he's doing. We can re-arrange an appointment with him for this afternoon if you like. What seems to be the problem?'

'My dog is vomiting,' she says.

'If that's the case, I think it might be better if I have a look at her rather than you waiting for Mr Singleton,' I reply.

'Well, if it must be,' she says.

This isn't uncommon. Brian is frequently away and his clients are consistently unhappy having to see such a young vet, even if I have quite a luxurious beard and think I now look wise and old.

'When did she start vomiting?' I ask, and am told it started the previous day.

'Did she vomit food or froth?' I ask.

'A balloon. She vomited a balloon,' the owner answers.

'That's odd,' I say, and the dog's owner explains that her dog loves carrying things in her mouth, and when her daughter tried to get an unused red balloon out of her mouth, the dog, not wanting to give up its possession, simply swallowed it.

'Is she still vomiting?' I ask.

'No. But she's not herself,' the owner replies.

I examine the dog, Honey, a three-year-old, and find nothing amiss.

'Has she had any diarrhoea?' I ask, and am told that she hasn't.

'Dogs have a sensitive vomiting reflex. If they eat anything unusual they vomit it back up, and that often ends the problem. I don't think we have to do anything right now.'

'But she's very subdued. She's not right,' the owner says. 'Should she have an X-ray?'

'Not at this stage. Why not offer her some of her regular food, and if she's not eating or seems to remain subdued I can see her again. You should see the red balloon in her poop tomorrow.'

I could see the owner was convinced something was still wrong. I worried I was missing it.

The next day brought another new experience. Among the morning appointments was an emergency, a seven-month-old Jack Russell-type dog named Rabbit, barking hysterically. He'd had a seizure at home, recovered quickly but now, as well as non-stop barking, he had twitching eyelids and muscle tremors. I injected him with ACP, a potent sedative, and after a few minutes he relaxed a little, although his eyelids continued to jerk and his muscles shake.

My first thought was post-distemper brain inflammation, a grave prognosis. I checked his medical records, and Rabbit had been vaccinated, by me, four months previously, so distemper was unlikely to be the cause. I asked how his bowels were, and was told he had had diarrhoea for several days and that he might have vomited. Now that he was relaxed and it was possible to examine him, I saw that his gum colour was excellent, but there was something else. There were flakes of grey paint in his mouth.

'Does he chew on anything?' I ask

'He's the most destructive dog I've ever had,' his owner, a blue-stockinged woman in a white blouse buttoned to her neck, probably only in her early forties but looking far older, answers. We all make instant judgements, and mine was that this woman was dead from the neck down.

'What does he chew?' I ask.

'Toys. Furniture. Doors. Baseboards. What *doesn't* he chew,' she replies.

'Does he chew through the paint?'

'Right down to the wood.'

'Do you know if there's any old paint on the doors or baseboards?' Rabbit's owner explains that the house she lives in is over 200 years old and has been repainted many times.

I excuse myself and interrupt Brian, who was consulting next door.

'Do you think Jean Shanks can check lead levels in blood?' I ask.

'Yes, and if you have a lead poisoning case there's calcium EDTA downstairs. Give it subcutaneously. Pat will calculate how much. Who is it?' Brian asks, and I tell him Rabbit Abbott.

'Mrs Abbott is a senior member of the Queen's household,' Brian says.

I send the blood sample by taxi to Jean Shanks on Harley Street, and feel very proud of myself when I learn that Rabbit did have lead poisoning and, I like to say, had been poisoned by the royal family.

I spent part of lunchtime at the RCVS library, fingering through the card indexes, looking for published papers on pain management in dogs. Some index drawers contained cards filed according to medical conditions. There were over a hundred references for 'Pancreatitis' but only four for 'Pain'. It seemed it wasn't a topic that was written about. I asked Miss Horder, the wonderfully named Head Librarian, for her advice, and she suggested I review the cards for 'Orthopaedic Surgery', as pain management might be mentioned in these scientific papers. She told me she would ask for a search at the British Library and get some reprints on inter-library loan.

Brian let me leave early that afternoon so that I could visit Keith's surgery on Kynance Mews to see it in operation. I only have six appointments to see after lunch, and one was Honey, the vomiting Golden Retriever from the previous day. When I saw the dog's name on the afternoon day sheet, I knew I was missing something.

'Hello. She's still not right,' the owner explains.

'Mr Singleton is here this afternoon if you'd like to see him,' I say.

'Yes, I know. I was offered an appointment with him, but as I've started with you I thought it was best to continue with you.'

'Is she still vomiting?' I ask.

'No.'

'Is she eating normally?'

'Yes.'

'Are her stools normal?'

'Yes, they are.'

'Has she passed the balloon yet?'

'Yes, she has.'

'And what's not right about her?'

'I can't put my finger on it,' she says, as she strokes her dog's head, 'but I know my dog and she's not right. She's not happy.'

'What's she doing to make you know she's not happy?'

'Look at her. She's subdued,' Honey's owner says. 'At home she either lies in her bed or goes under the kitchen table, where she has taken her toys. Sometimes she moans, and it sounds as if something is hurting her.'

'Has she been spayed?' I ask, and am told that she hasn't.

'When was she last in season?' She had a season around six weeks previously, I'm told. I examine her and feel something I missed the previous day. Her nipples are enlarged and she has starting to produce milk.'

'Aha,' I exclaim triumphantly. 'You're absolutely right she's not right, but this has nothing to do with her swallowing the balloon, and she's going to get better without our help.'

'What do you mean?' the blonde asks in a questioning but innocent way.

'She's simply finding it rough being a woman,' I say. 'After each season, dogs naturally go through a hormonal pregnancy. Whether they're pregnant or not they produce the hormone of pregnancy, progesterone. That hormone can do many things, including making her behave in a subdued way, stimulating her to mother her toys, encouraging her to find a safe den, like under your kitchen table. Honey's in the middle of a normal false pregnancy.'

I'm concentrating on trying to ensure I'm making the right diagnosis, and it's obvious that this attractive woman is too concerned about her dog's well-being to see me as anything other than someone too young and inexperienced to know what he's talking about.

'It can't be as simple as that,' the woman says firmly. 'Are you sure?'

I give the dog another cursory examination.

'Yes, I am. And of course Mr Singleton is just next door if you'd like his opinion.'

Honey's owner declines the offer, and I head off to South Kensington and Keith's surgery.

The more central London surgeries I saw, the more I realised how spacious Brian's was. At first I had compared Pont Street to what I was familiar with in Canada, where all facilities were always on an extensive ground floor. Brian's building had a small footprint, but at least he had four floors of space to live and work in. John had a smaller footprint and three floors. Keith's mews house had an even smaller footprint and just two floors.

Keith, tall and fit, with a broad forehead, chiselled features and thick hair, reminded me of the film star Laurence Harvey in *The Charge of the Light Brigade*, but rather than appearing in smart imperial uniform he was in a floor-length green operating gown inviting his next client from the tiny waiting area into his examination room. Both rooms are not much wider than I am tall. Two cats rest contentedly on open circular stairs to the first floor.

'Hello, Bruce. Have a look around,' he says, and his receptionist suggests I go through the door behind her. This leads to a combined kennel, storage and X-ray room, and a door from there leads to the operating room. Another door opens to his examination room and then back to the reception area. Somehow he has squeezed four rooms into a space no larger than fifteen by twenty feet. Up an open stairway on the first floor is a lounge, kitchen and two bedrooms. Keith is taller than I am, and I'm a bit over six foot. I marvel that he can work in such a tiny place.

My clockwise tour of his premises brings me to his examination room, where, as Keith examines another dog that has been waiting in reception, his RANA writes down his observations in the dog's medical record.

'Heart rate 132. Lungs clear. Cap refill delayed. Heavy plaque. Mild splenic enlargement.'

Keith turns his eyes to the dog's owner. 'When was the last time she vomited?' and when he is told an hour previously, his RANA also writes that down.

At Pont Street we had appointments every fifteen minutes. By having someone take notes for him, Keith could see six cases each hour, 50 per cent more than I did. Working on his own with a staff of three, his caseload was virtually the same as the one that Brian and I shared.

I stayed as he saw his last five patients. Rather than the intercom system we had to use because our consulting rooms were on the floor above the waiting room, Keith was more informal, escorting a client out and inviting the next one in. At Brian's we always used surnames, but with some of his clients Keith welcomes them by their given names. One woman kisses him hello and he seems a bit taken aback when she does. He is thorough with his examinations. I liked his suggestions for treatments. I think he is the type of guy I'd be happy to take my dog or cat to. In fact, that's what I've done in the fifty years since, when I've wanted another mind to mull over a problem. I'd chanced upon a future friend, another slender tendril to root me to Britain.

After the last client leaves, and while his staff make the place tidy and finish the day's book-keeping, we go upstairs, followed by the cats. A Springer spaniel that has been snoozing on the sofa gets off, stretches herself and walks over to greet us. Keith strokes his dog, lights a cigar and pours me a glass of wine.

'That's Maude,' he explains, nodding towards the Springer. 'Are you busy at Pont Street?' he asks, and although it is a simple question, I have no point of reference as I've never worked anywhere else. So I explain that appointments are usually fully booked in all the allotted slots, but seeing how he sees six people each hour, it doesn't seem anywhere near as busy as his surgery does.

'Are you busy here?' I ask, and Keith, sitting on an office chair, absent-mindedly tickling Maude behind her ears, puffs on his cigar and gives a slight nod.

'Do you go on many home visits?' I ask.

'That's the luxury of the multi-man practice,' he smiles, then he adds, 'Are you going to take up Frank's offer?'

That surprises me.

'How do you know Frank offered me a job?'

Keith just smiles and puffs on his cigar.

One of the cats, a tabby and white, leaps onto my lap, curls itself into a tight ball and dozes off.

'She's a bit of a flirt,' Keith says.

'They're yours?' I ask.

'Yes. Maude's a working Springer. The cats arrived by accident.' I ask what he means, and he explains they had been brought in to be put down.

'Together?' I ask.

'No,' he replies then, after another puff on his cigar, shrugging his shoulders, adds, 'What do you do?'

'Got anything planned this evening?' I ask, and Keith explains he and his wife are going to friends for dinner. Although I'd met him several times, I didn't know he was married.

It had started to drizzle, yet again, when I left Kynance Mews. When you feel alone, London's drab, clammy climate infiltrates deep into your being. Rather than walking back to Pont Street I took the Circle Line, getting off at Sloane Square. I saw that a new play, *Lulu*, was on at the Royal Court Theatre, so rather than go back to my flat to dine on my own I bought a ticket. There was time to grab a bowl of stew at the nearby Chelsea Stockpot then watch the play, the story of either a libertine or a naïf – I couldn't decide which – who has sex with everyone. The actress who played Lulu spent most of the evening either undressed or being undressed.

After the play I walked back to Pont Street. I hadn't heard from Rose for weeks and suddenly had a thought she was back but simple avoiding me. I walked past the surgery, over to her

mews, and although there were no lights on, I still knocked on
the door, hoping she was there. She wasn't.

On Wednesday the weather improved. I awoke to dawn
sunshine and my weekly morning ride on Euripides was terrific.
By now we understood each other so well I was allowed to take
him through the traffic around Hyde Park Corner without
being led by a groom. I can't tell you what a difference it makes
seeing Hyde Park from horseback. That seemingly insignificant
increased height gives you a totally different and fresh perspective, and on a sunny spring day, with the trees in blossom and
spring flowers radiating, it was intoxicating. The night before I
hated London. Now I loved it.

My first patient was a three-year-old blue roan Cocker
spaniel accompanied by his owner, an attractive but brusque
brunette in her early thirties and her eight-year-old curly-
haired, sombre and sad-looking son. The dog had been dragging its bum on the ground and she thought it had worms. At
veterinary college the fact that dogs have territory-marking
anal sacs may have been mentioned, but if it had been I missed
it. In my first year at Brian's I learned that not only do dogs
have anal sacs, but that anal sac problems pay for vet's holi-
days. They get blocked, abscessed, need emptying or syringing,
even removing.

'You know, Sally is William's best friend,' Sally's rather over-
bearing owner explains as I lift the dog's tail and confirm that
the sacs are impacted.

William stares at the floor. He doesn't say anything.

'I grew up with Scotties and Yorkshire terriers,' I say to
William, but he remains mute.

'William, say something to the vet,' his mother commands,
and I can see from the way he moves his feet that William feels
uncomfortable.

I ask Sally's owner to hold her dog's front-end firmly as I lift the Cocker's tail and with cotton wool in my hand squeeze the anal sacs empty. 'Yuck!' I say a bit theatrically, in William's direction.

I lift Sally off the table and put her on the floor, where she immediately licks her bum. William is watching.

'William, I know what she's thinking. Once she's finished she's going to want to lick your face.' He smiles.

As I write on Sally's medical record, 'AGE', the shorthand I use for 'anal glands emptied', not looking at William, I say, 'I had a dog named Angus, and we'd sit together and watch ducks floating on the lake. We didn't have to talk to each other. We knew exactly what each other was thinking. Without having to say anything.'

After a short pause William says, 'Me too.'

His mother looks at me with an astonished expression.

I explain to her that if Sally starts dragging her bottom again, the sacs will need emptying once more and the RANAs can do that.

As they leave the room, William's owner turns and mouths silently, 'He never says anything.'

I follow them out into the hallway, and as they walk down the stairs say, 'William, I thought it was fun to write to friends, telling them why I loved Angus.'

Pat had told me that the elderly woman bringing in her Persian cat that morning was a dowager duchess. Although the cat was only eight years old, it was losing weight and drinking more water than previously. 'She's spending so many pennies,' I'm told, a comment that when I first heard it I needed one of the staff to interpret for me.

The cat's owner is charming, a soft-spoken, elegant woman with a gentleness of spirit and a refined beauty. She has magnificent grey hair piled in a luxuriant but restless pompadour. We should, of course, treat all people as equals, but her inner beauty made me want to do everything possible to diagnose and treat her cat's condition. Drusilla was dehydrated and I admitted her for the day, to give intravenous fluids, take a blood sample to check her kidney function and, because her kidneys felt large and rough, to X-ray her abdomen.

We admitted another patient that morning, Max, a German Shepherd with an open bleeding tumour on his hind leg, and between these extra procedures and operations already booked we were going to be hard pressed to finish before afternoon appointments began at 3 pm.

Pat ensured that Annabelle worked hard in her first week. With Pat giving instructions, Annabelle acted as theatre nurse.

Brian had invested in a new piece of biochemistry equipment called a Unimeter, with which we could do simple blood tests at the surgery without the delay that happened when samples were sent by post – which we still couldn't do because of a months-long postal strike. Brian had bought the equipment, in part because it seemed as if the postal strike would go on forever.

A quick X-ray of Drusilla's belly confirms that both her kidneys are enlarged and cystic, full of round, fluid-filled pockets. After putting her on an intravenous drip and taking a blood sample, we move on to two cats to be sterilised. The anaesthetic we had been clinically trialling, CT1341, we had a large supply of thanks to Glaxo. The cats had been given sedatives and atropine,* to reduce saliva before I went

---

* Atropine is an 'anticholinesterase inhibitor' that reduces bronchial secretions. That means less saliva in the mouth that might accidentally get down the windpipe when an animal is anaesthetised. (It was also used as the antidote when pets were poisoned by organophosphate flea sprays.)

downstairs, and are ready for surgery. Pat shows Annabelle how to raise a vein in the front leg, which she does, then how to clip and prepare the belly of the female for surgery. While I operate, Pat does a 'blood urea nitrogen' or 'BUN' test on Drusilla's blood using the Unimeter.

'Do cat's ears go red when they're anaesthetised?' Annabelle asks.

I look at the cat's ears and see they are red – deep red.

'Give them a feel,' I ask her.

'They feel hot and puffy.'

'No, they don't usually go red. It must be something about this cat.'

'Drusilla's BUN is 42,' Pat reports. 'With this reagent it should be under 10.'

We know that the high BUN, together with the cystic kidneys seen on X-ray and her pronounced dehydration, mean that she has 'polycystic kidney disease', a condition seen frequently in Persians but rarely in other breeds or moggies and for which little can be done. The cat will die within months.

Annabelle successfully raises the vein on the tom cat without Pat's help, and while I quickly castrate it, she says, 'Now that we're decimal, why is Mr Singleton still charging in guineas?'

'Well, my dear,' Pat replies, 'simply because a guinea is five new pence more than a pound and *a guinea, please* sounds better than *one pound and five new pence, please*. Do you think he should hire girls in boaters and blue sashes like Harrods does to explain the decimal system to our clients?'

'It sounds so toffee-nosed,' Annabelle says.

'Well, we can see who you'll be voting for when you're old enough,' Pat adds somewhat curtly.

'If you think I'd vote Labour, I voted for Edward Heath and I'd fire all the postmen. Imagine! Asking for a 20 per cent pay rise and selfishly going on strike for so long. Nobody gets a 20 per cent pay rise!'

'You're not old enough to vote, love!' Pat says. 'You're still eighteen.'

'I'll be nineteen in two months and don't forget, voting age was reduced last year, in time for me to vote.'

Pat turns to me. 'Well, Brucie, how did you know that Annabelle bats for the right team?'

We move on to the last proper op, the German Shepherd. The tumour is large and open, like a four-inch-wide explosion of red, raw cauliflower on its right hip. It too has been given its sedative while I operate on the cats. Once more, under Pat's supervision, Annabelle raises the vein, prepares the dog's skin for surgery and lays out my surgical instruments.

While I scrub up, I ask her why she was working in Harrods' pet department.

'I've wanted to work with animals ever since my mother told me about Laika, the space dog,' she replies. 'I was four or five years old at the time. My mother told me because she thought it was amazing that a dog travelled to space, but I thought it was horrible that that poor dog died up there all alone. Did you watch the Apollo landing on the moon last month? Can you imagine how horrible it was for that poor dog to be in a space capsule with nothing to eat or drink and to die all alone?'

'I can,' I say. 'And I don't believe them when they say they euthanised Laika the way they say they did. She starved to death. Or froze to death, if they couldn't keep the temperature up.' In fact, fifty years later, when the Russians finally revealed truths about their space programme, it was learned that Laika boiled to death shortly after the space capsule reached orbit.

The operation went smoothly. Although the mass was mobile and on the surface of the skin, I did a wide and deep excision. Professor Levene would tell me by the end of the week whether it was a one-off haemangioma or a far nastier malignant haemangiosarcoma. It was a tight fit, pulling the skin together, and I sutured two lengths of rubber tubing on either side of the incision, as Brian did, with mattress stitches through the tubing to avoid tearing tension from individual stitches. Because of the size of the tumour, I arranged with his owner that Max stay the night. If it had been any other day, Max would have been taken by Brian to Limpsfield for surgery, followed by a week of hospitalisation, but it was Wednesday and Brian was already there, working his way through his operations. I'd check on Max downstairs overnight. In the meantime there was one final procedure, a dental on a Yorkshire terrier. It was almost 3 pm, so I anaesthetised the dog and told Pat I might want her to do the dental. But when I look in the dog's mouth, every single tooth root is rotten. The mildest touch of dental forceps is all that's needed to remove every single tooth.

'How can someone let things get that bad?' Annabelle asks.

'Because some people love their dogs too much,' Pat replies.

'Go on,' I say.

'Well, Mr Singleton has been after Rufus's owner to have his teeth done for over three years now, but she's refused because she was worried about the anaesthetic. She only brought him in now because he can't hold food in his mouth, it is so painful. Poor thing. In a fortnight he'll be acting like a puppy.'

'But without any teeth, how will he eat?' Annabelle asks.

'Comfortably!' Pat beams back. 'Mind you, without his canines his tongue will hang out like a little pink kazoo.'

Max recovered from his anaesthetic just before I finished the dental, and he started barking and howling. He wanted out of his kennel. It was just after 3 pm and I double-stepped up the stairs from the basement to the first floor, noticing the pretty blonde woman with the Golden Retriever in the waiting room as I passed by. She was back yet again. What was I missing?

With Max barking incessantly downstairs and Honey the Golden Retriever with something still wrong with her in the waiting room, I didn't concentrate on my first patient. Honey was next and Brian wasn't there, so I didn't have the pragmatic escape valve I was so grateful for and frequently used of, 'Brian, if you have a minute, can you come in and have a look at this?'

Honey leads her owner up the stairs and into the consulting room. The dog must think this is her new daily routine. When they enter the consulting room, I notice for the first time that they are remarkably similar, two tousle-haired, natural blondes with very attractive curves and winning smiles.

'Hello again. I know you think it silly, but I've come back just to make sure that Honey is perfectly fine and just enduring her hormones. Mind you, I know *exactly* how she feels!'

'You know how she feels?' I ask.

'Hormones! I get the most splitting migraines when I have my period.'

Two things. First of all, I notice that Honey's owner is actually looking at me, probably for the first time, and she's smiling, and she has the most enormous black eyelashes on all four eyelids and are they actually fluttering at me? Second, she's given me possibly more information than I want to know. I examine the dog once more and find nothing amiss, other than her active mammary glands.

'Eating. Drinking. Peeing. Pooping. All okay?' I ask.

'Yes, other than her lying under the kitchen table and mothering her toys, she seems fine.'

As I finish examining her, the dog gives me a lick. I give her a tickle behind her ears and she presses her head into my chest, asking me to continue.

'Dogs!' her owner says, still smiling and fluttering those amazing eyelashes. 'Just like us. Love a cuddle.'

As the afternoon progressed, Max continued barking. At 4 pm I suggested to Brenda that as Max would be staying the night, to take him upstairs to my flat and see if he was less stressed there. It worked. As soon as he was out of a kennel and had a sofa he could climb onto, he settled down. Brenda provided him with a water bowl and I would feed him later.

After the afternoon appointments finished, I took Drusilla to her home, two minutes away in Cadogan Place. The sun had shone all day and the early evening light had turned the square a rich, magical golden. The dowager duchess answered the door.

'I am so pleased and grateful to you,' she says. 'Now do come in. I have some questions for you.'

She turns and walks down her hallway into her elegant lounge, stopping once to steady herself with her hand against a wall.

'Do have a drink with me.'

I see she is drinking whisky from a cut crystal decanter and her stopping to lean against the wall isn't because of age or frailty.

I open Drusilla's wicker cat carrier and she whizzes out, rubs herself against the corner of the sofa and disappears from the room. I assume she is heading for her litter tray.

'Yes, thank you very much,' I say, and the dowager duchess pours me a very, very large Scotch.

'Water?' she asks. I nod, and she adds a little.

'Thank you ever so much for taking such good care of Drusilla.'

She pulls her chair over to me, close enough for our knees to almost touch. Her woollen suit is immaculate, a cream top, buttoned to the neck with large black buttons, and a straight skirt. Around her neck is a single strand of pearls and on her fingers several gold rings, all with different-sized rubies, diamonds and small pearls. She leans forward, grasps my arm with her hand and looks straight at me. Her eyes are warm and welcoming but also rheumy.

'I find Drusilla's condition quite confusing and medical jargon is beyond me, so think of me as your mother and tell me the prognosis.'

'Her condition is not unexpected for a Persian cat,' I say. 'Within the breed there's a genetic predisposition for the kidneys to become cystic at a relatively early age. The cystic tissue has no ability to filter, so as cystic masses develop, filtration diminishes. That's what's happening with Drusilla. We did an in-house blood test and her blood urea nitrogen is over four times above the upper limit of normal. The intravenous fluids she's had today have flushed out a lot of waste from her body, but I'm afraid her kidneys just don't have much viable tissue left. That's why she's drinking more and that's why she's losing weight. She's losing protein in her urine, so she's finding the energy she needs in her own fat and muscles.'

The dowager duchess leans closer to me and looks straight into my eyes.

'I'm so glad I'm not your mother,' she says with a wry smile.

I change direction. 'In simple terms, although she's only eight years old, it's as if her kidneys are twenty years old. They're failing and I'm afraid I can't do anything to make them healthy again. She's perfectly comfortable but her end will come sometime this year.'

'Thank you, Dr Fogle,' she says. 'I appreciate your honesty.' Then she adds, 'My son could learn a lesson from you.'

I decide it is better not to ask why.

'Another drink?' she asks, but I am still nursing the first one.

'My son has the most dreadful taste in women,' she continues.

'He is enamoured with scarlet. Is it not astonishing that some men cannot see through the motives of women?'

I decide to be non-committal.

'Well, some of us follow our heads, some our hearts and I guess some of us follow our trousers.'

'Then you must know my son!' she replies. 'And he has neither a head nor a heart.'

She continues, 'After my husband died, I hoped my daughter would talk sense into my son. Daughters are so sensible. Do you have sisters, Dr Fogle?'

I tell her I have one, much younger than me.

'Does she live here? You are such a nice young man. Perhaps you could bring her here the next time you visit. I can ensure my son will be here.'

'I'm afraid she's at university in Canada,' I explain.

'Pity,' she says.

I felt uncomfortable with her telling me about her sadness with her son. Ten years later, after organising an international meeting called the Human Companion Animal Bond and listening to, among others, the psychiatrists I had invited to give talks, I have a better understanding of why she shared her melancholy with me. But there was also another lesson for me. She was a genuine upper-class woman, yet she was asking if I had an available sister for her son to meet. Could it be that in some way the upper class could be classless?

'Pedigree Petfoods has something new called Nephritis Diet,' I say. 'It's for dogs, but drop in tomorrow and pick up a tin. If Drusilla eats it, it might be good for her kidneys.'

That was rotten advice. I was still thinking that cats are dogs that miaow. They aren't, and their nutritional needs are quite different. A dog can survive quite nicely eating cat food but the reverse isn't true.

I excused myself and returned to the surgery. Over an hour had passed and the RANAs had gone home, but there was a letter addressed to me on the reception desk. Max was quiet. I picked up the letter, walked up the two flights of stairs and opened the door to my flat. A tornado had swept through it. My bed had been stripped. The sofa cushions were on the floor. So were my records and my books.

Max, in his Elizabethan collar so he wouldn't chew his surgical site, was sitting on the floor looking embarrassed.

'Jesus, Max! Can't you ever relax?' I thunder.

He gets up and walks slowly to me, with his head down.

'Well, you don't need this on when I'm here,' I tell him, and I take off his Elizabethan collar and sit down to read the letter. As soon as I am on the sofa, Max comes over and puts a forepaw on my lap and looks straight into my eyes.

'Okay. You're handsome,' I say, and give his chest a rub. As I do so he puts his other forepaw on my lap.

'Easy, Max,' I say. 'That's a precious part of my anatomy.' He keeps looking at me, this massive-headed, warm brown-eyed, shiny-haired beast.

'You're a good looking guy,' I say. 'Why aren't you noble like this when you're on your own?' He leans forward, gives my face a lick and surreptitiously puts a hind leg on the sofa. In another instant his final leg is up and he is on my lap, where he sits, looking out at the room. He weighs a ton, but I feel comfortable with him there. I like it.

Poor guy, I think. He hasn't a clue what's happening. All he knows is he goes somewhere strange, falls asleep, wakes up and nothing is familiar. He's completely discombobulated but he thinks at least there's a human here. I'll protect him.

I feel curiously comfortable with Max on my lap and I open the envelope. There are two papers in it. The first note says:

Dear Dr Fogle,
Thank you for being so kind to William today. I'm sure
you saw we have a problem with him although we don't
know exactly what it is. This is a letter that he wrote
when we returned home. He has asked me to give it to
you.
   With sincere thanks,
   Belinda Tomlinson

I open William's note. It is short and written in large but legible
writing.

My dog means somebody nice and quiet to be with. She
doesn't say do like my mother or don't like my father or
stop like my brother. My dog Sally and me sit together
and I like her and she likes me. The end.

'Brucie, you have a special visitor today,' Pat trumpets when I
come downstairs the next day.

'He doesn't get it, does he,' Annabelle adds.

'Well, let me see what's on your day sheet. You've got a goldfish swimming on its side, a lame dog, a macaw with overgrown
nails, a dog finding it hard to pee, a cat finding it hard to pee
and, Annabelle, look at this, there's a Miss Foster with her
Golden Retriever Honey booked in at 11.45 am. I wonder
whatever she might be coming in for?'

'Is that the dog I've seen every day this week?' I ask.

'Bingo! You're such an observant young vet,' Pat replies.

'That dog is absolutely fine. What is it with her owner?' I
exclaim.

'Well, you'll just have to find out,' Pat says.

I didn't have any good suggestions for the goldfish owner, my
first client of the day. My hunch was a problem with the swim

bladder, but I knew nothing about fish medical conditions then and still don't.

The lame dog was a simple diagnosis and treatment. Barrington, a lurcher, had leapt over a wall in Battersea Park, not realising that the far side was much lower than the near one. He had no difficulty getting up the stairs to my consulting room but limped into the room, favouring his left foreleg. When I flexed his shoulder I felt nothing broken or torn but he winced. I wrote out a prescription for prednisone, a steroid anti-inflammatory, for the nurses to dispense, explaining to his owner that he would drink and urinate more while on the pills. Today I'd use a non-steroid anti-inflammatory rather than a steroid. I explained that he should have no exercise until the following Monday and if he was still lame he should be returned for an X-ray. I carried him down the stairs so he didn't have to bear weight on his sore shoulder.

'Hello, Dr Fogle. I am Martin Hensler,' the macaw owner says as he offers me his hand, which I shake. His macaw is on his shoulder. Nine months on and I still wasn't paying much attention to my clients, but with his deep tan, imposing height, high cheekbones, immaculately cut, long wavy hair and tailored Harris tweed suit, he was ruggedly good looking, probably in his late thirties.

'Mr Singleton see our dogs but he tell me you have zoo experience and suggest it is best for you to cut claws.' The man has an accent that I can't place but soon learn is Hungarian.

'He is okay. Don't bite,' the owner explains.

I move my downturned hand slowly towards the bird's feet on the man's shoulder and the macaw instantly hits it with his beak.

'Unless he don't know you,' the owner adds, giving me a proud grin. 'But he is okay. Clipping claws no problem. Is just I need someone to help and Sir John in New York. Other birds okays.'

'Do you have more macaws?' I ask.

'Yes, many birds. Small and large. Mostly parrot. Sir John has aviary for them. I put bird on table then hold beak and you cut claws.'

As the owner bends down for the bird to step off his shoulder onto the table, I wonder who 'Sir John' is.

Martin, as I will soon know him, tickles the top of the big bird's head and it leans into his tickling. He puts his arm over the macaw in case it goes for me, and with its claws resting on the table I started clipping them.

'What's Sir John doing in New York?' I ask, hoping to get a clue about who he is from the answer.

'Is in New York directing Edward Albee play,' Martin answers.

The only knighted director I can think of is Sir John Gielgud, so I say, 'Not acting?' and Martin replies, 'No.'

Presto! Detective Fogle is right!

'I thought he was outstanding in *Home*,' I continue.

'You like *Home*? You know he is good in *Home* because he plays mixed-up man and is really mixed-up man. He doesn't understand script, so isn't acting. Is same with Ralph Richardson.'

Home by David Storey, at the Royal Court Theatre in Sloane Square, set in a mental asylum, was one of the first plays I saw when I arrived in London. I'd seen Sir John Gielgud in a play with Vivien Leigh in Toronto in 1966. Now, here I am clipping his macaw's claws. I have also given Elizabeth Taylor and Richard Burton's dogs pedicures. Part of me finds all of this exciting. Another part of me finds it rather bizarre, but the biggest part of me implicitly understands that what I am learning is that people may be famous, adored for their unique abilities, but underneath the fame they are the same as everyone else.

'He is back May. Perhaps you tell him then how much you like *Home*,' Martin adds, as he shakes my hand once more and leaves the room.

The dog having difficulty peeing was an avuncular nine-year-old male yellow Labrador.

'I'm sure it's prostatic hyperplasia,' his owner explains.* 'I've tested his urine and it's normal. I'd manually examine his prostate, but I don't want to hurt him so it's over to you.'

I look at Charmer's medical record and see his owner's address is on Harley Street. He must be a doctor.

'We use Jean Shanks for our urine cultures,' I say and his eyes light up.

'The very best. I didn't think you did such things with dogs.'

Charmer was a big dog and I have long and lean fingers so, as with other dogs, he didn't resent a rubber-gloved finger fidgeting with his prostate. It was enormous.

'This should shrink it,' I say, taking a bottle of 'Tardak' from the shelf.

'Delmidinone, a by-product of the Pill,' I continue.

Charmer's owner examines the bottle.

'Delmidinone acetate, from Syntex. I'm not familiar with it. Did Syntex develop the Pill?'

'At university I heard a lecture from Carl Djerassi, one of the Pill's inventors, and he says they did.'

'What was his story?' Charmer's owner asks.

'An American chemist moved to Mexico around the time I was born, set up Syntex and went looking for plants with substances that could be degraded to cortisone and progesterone. At that time progesterone for medical use was still being

---

* Prostatic hyperplasia: enlargement of the prostate gland.

collected from pregnant mares' serum and bulls' balls. He heard that healers in Oaxaca used fermented Mexican yams to treat aching joints or induce abortion, and developed a technique to cheaply convert yam steroids to cortisone and progesterone. The Pill manufacturers get their hormones from Syntex. This was one of their dead ends. It prevented women from ovulating but put them off sex, so it got shelved. Ten years later they went back to it, thinking it must be good for something and it is, shrinking Charmer's prostate, and his sex drive too. The insert says, *For the treatment of canine satyriasis.*'

I give Charmer an injection.

'He should pee easier within a few days. If he does, I'll give another injection in a week or so. If he doesn't, we should X-ray to make sure it's no more complicated than benign prostatic hyperplasia, then castrate.'

'That would be a tough sell with my patients,' Charmer's owner says.

'What would you do?' I ask.

'Resect the prostate. It can be done through the urethra,' I'm told, and I explain I wish it were that easy in dogs but to get to the prostate is extremely difficult and might even involve cracking open the pelvic bone.

The cat having difficulty urinating was more problematic. Ginger had been able to pee with difficulty when the appointment was made the day before, but now he was completely blocked and in terrible pain. When I palpated his abdomen his bladder felt as large and as hard as a cricket ball. His plaintive howling was extremely distressing.

I call Brenda to help, and for immediate relief stick a needle through his abdominal wall into his bladder and using a 50 ml glass syringe remove over 150 ml of bloody urine. It's a dramatic procedure that provides immediate pain relief but the hard part follows, getting a catheter through the grit in Ginger's urethra into his bladder. Brenda takes him downstairs and gives him a sedative in preparation for catheterising.

I want to get straight down to him but there is the final morning appointment with Honey and her owner.

'It's getting to feel just like home here,' Honey's bouncy owner breathes as they enter my consulting room. She's smiling at me in the same way she did on the last visit.

Her dog is smiling too, but my mind is on Ginger.

'Listen, I'm an actress and I'm in a play right now, and I wonder whether you might like some tickets to it, you know, as a thank you for taking such good care of Honey.'

She turns and looks, somewhat theatrically I think, at her dog.

I think what a lovely thing to do, and now, looking at her more closely, rather than at her dog, I see an attractive, gentle, almost embarrassed face. And big hair. Big, big hair.

'That's really nice. I love the theatre. Is this your first play?'

'Well, I've been an actress for some time now,' she says. 'Mostly films but several West End plays. It's nice you'd like to come. How many tickets would you like?'

'One would be fine, thank you.'

She smiles softly. All the while Honey sits by her side.

'Is there any night that is best for you?' she asks, and as I have no plans this evening I say that would be good.

'Oh, dear. That's soon. I'll have to see that the house seats are still available. If you don't hear from me this afternoon, they are. Go to the box office and ask for Mr Lowenstein's seats. Give them your name and tell them Julia Foster has made arrangements.'

'Thanks. By the way, which theatre should I go to?'

'The Royal Court. I'm in a play called *Lulu*.'

She offers me her hand and leaves, and I race down to Ginger, thinking, Royal Court, *Lulu*. Was she the actress I saw two nights earlier?

Ginger's blocked bladder was a challenge. There was a virtual epidemic of tom cats with blocked bladders in the early 1970s, a problem that was eventually traced back to their food. New dry foods on the market resulted in urine that was only just on the acidic side of neutral, which is 'pH 7'. In some cats, a urine pH over 6.5 increases the possibility of a cat making so many triple phosphate or 'struvite' crystals they cause a blockage. That's what Ginger had. When cat food makers realised the problem they reformulated their foods, but now some of these foods produced urine that was too acidic. If a cat's urine pH was less than 5.5 he might also block, but now with a different crystal called calcium oxalate.

Blocked bladders are much less common today, probably because cat-food makers finally got their balances right, but this was my first exposure to medical problems that were wholly our creation. In the following decades, I would see other medical problems caused by commercial foods, drugs, vaccines, anti-parasitic treatments, even seemingly innocent toys. I would learn to be sceptical about any claims that industries made about their products, sometimes to the point of disbelieving until proven otherwise. I would learn that less is often best, that the role of the vet is not to cure but to create circumstances in which the pet cures itself. In a gratifyingly large selection of situations, that involves no more than controlling pain and ensuring good hydration.

Brenda helped me anaesthetise Ginger, and using a new type of tom-cat catheter, a 'Jackson', I gradually got the catheter in. It takes patience, moving millimetres at a time, always back-flushing with, at that time, Walpole's solution, feeling the grit the catheter encounters in the urethra, identifying with the poor guy, imagining how dreadful it must feel. When Ginger's

urethra was free of grit and the catheter was safely into his
bladder, I sewed it in place. Brenda put an Elizabethan collar on
him so he wouldn't chew it out.

'It's Thursday, and we should keep him for at least two
days.'

'I'll come in over the weekend,' she says.

'That's okay,' I reply. 'I'll be here so I can check on him.'

After work I changed into my dark blue velvet suit, white
shirt with blue flowers and blue satin tie, grabbed the Scotch
egg I'd got from Express Dairy as a quick bite to eat, walked
down to the Royal Court, picked up my ticket from the box
office and took my seat. Best seat in the house. The seat beside
me was empty and I realised I could have asked for two if I'd
wanted, which I didn't, sort of. The actress is cute. I know she
is married – her dog had swallowed one of her daughter's
balloons – but even if Rose had been back, I still wanted to go
on my own.

The play is still gothic, still very Bertolt Brecht–Kurt Weill.
The audience give her a standing ovation at the curtain call, and
I am quite proud that of all of them I am the one who will see
her in her dressing room afterwards.

I've bought a couple of bunches of freesias from a Sloane
Square flower seller before the performance, and with those in
hand go around to the stage door, introduce myself and tell the
doorman that Miss Foster is expecting me. He tells me which
corridor to take and which room to go to, and as I approach I
hear loud, laughing voices.

The door is open but I knock anyway, and my client emerges
through the crowd in her tiny room, in a clinging, form-
revealing satin dressing gown.

*Whoops. I've come to Marilyn Monroe's dressing room by
accident.*

'Oh, it's so sweet of you to come. How did you like the play?

Come in and meet my friends!' Julia, as I now felt comfortable calling her, takes my hand and walks me in.

'This is my best friend, the playwright and critic Frank Marcus and his wife Jackie. Frank, Bruce is a vet.'

'A vet, eh?' Frank says. 'Do you think you can tame this animal?' Everyone laughs. I don't know what to say. Or do.

'This is my producer, Oscar Lowenstein, and his friend Joel Grey from New York. You probably know that Joel has won Tony Awards for *Cabaret* and *George M!*. He's visiting London.'

'Don't forget. I also played Arthur Kipps in *Half a Sixpence*,' Joel adds.

'But Tommy played Arthur Kipps in New York,' Julia says.

'I replaced Tommy. And I replaced Anthony Newley in *Stop the World*.'

'Imagine. You have *almost* worked with so many of my leading men,' Julia says.

'Joel has just finished filming *Cabaret* and I wager he's in for an Academy Award,' Oscar Lowenstein interjects.

I don't know what to say to all of this. There is an artificiality to their conversation and I don't know how to join in. So I say, 'Does your husband pick you up from the theatre each night?'

'We've been separated for some time,' she replies.

I offer her the flowers I have brought.

'Oh, that is so thoughtful of you!' and she gives me a kiss on my cheek. 'Do have some champagne,' and she gives me a champagne glass and fills it.

I scan her dressing room and it has more flowers in it than my father's flower shop.

'Lots of flowers,' I say.

Julia looks around her room. 'Oh yes, I have a fan who sends flowers each night. I met him at the stage door and told him he really mustn't send any more, and he was so crestfallen. I said he mustn't because I had nothing left to put them in. The next day more fresh flowers arrived from Harrods, this time with twelve vases!' She giggles then turns to Frank's wife Jackie.

'Jackie, it is so good to see you. I'm sure that all of you will want to have a meal together and talk theatre.'

'Right everybody! Drink up!' Jackie says. 'Follow me and give Julia some peace.' She kisses Julia goodbye, as do all the other visitors and finally we are alone.

'How's Honey?' I ask.

'Still hormonal, as you said she would be. Please. Sit down,' she says and I do. 'So tell me. What do you think of the play?'

That is a difficult question to answer. I didn't want to say that I liked the sex but hated the play, so I said, 'How do you interpret it?'

'Well, Frank Wedekind, the author, describes me as a wild, beautiful animal. That's why my friend Frank asked if you could tame me.'

'I lost track of who's who in the play,' I say, really just to make conversation.

'Well, there's Dr Schön, the rich publisher who rescues me from the streets, educates me and beds me,' she explains. 'Then there's Dr Goll, who he passes me on to. Dr Goll has my portrait painted by Schwarz, who I seduce, then Dr Goll finds out I've seduced Schwarz and drops dead from a heart attack. Then I marry Schwarz but remain Dr Schön's mistress. Then Dr Schön tells Schwarz about my licentious past and Schwarz slits his throat. That gets us through the first two acts.'

'What did you think when you first read the script?' I ask.

'It was for the Nottingham Playhouse and to be fair I didn't think it was possible to portray so much sex on stage. But it was, and we transferred here and from here we're transferring to the Apollo on Shaftesbury Avenue. Now, in Act Three, with the help of Dr Schön's son Alwa, who is also infatuated by me, I get a job dancing in a review, but Dr Schön still lusts after me and calls off his engagement to his fiancée Charlotte. I marry him but have sex with his son, my father, a circus performer and a lesbian countess. So Dr Schön gives me a gun to shoot myself but instead of shooting myself I shoot him, even though, deep inside I love him. Are you following? So I go to prison but with the help of my lesbian lover Countess Geschwitz, I escape from prison, go to London and eventually get my comeuppance at the hands of Jack the Ripper. So what do you make of it all? Am I a tart or taken advantage of?'

I really don't know what to say, so I proffer, 'You probably have a much better idea than I have. What do you think?'

'I think I am a man's fantasy woman. I love sex and have it with anyone. Every man finds what he wants in me but none of them think or care whether I have any needs. The portrait Schwarz painted of me, as Pierrot, is important. In commedia dell'arte Pierrot is comic but also naïve, even pathetic. That portrait is supposed to remind the audience that at heart I'm completely vulnerable. That's how I play her.'

'But also oversexed,' I add. 'The play's really intense. How do you leave her behind after each night's performance?'

'Whatever part I play, I find it impossible to leave the character at the stage door. As long as I play a role, that character becomes part of me.'

I wonder what she's like on a date, I think to myself.

'Do you go straight home from the theatre?' I ask.

'I usually eat after I come off, but it's Parents' Day at my daughter's nursery tomorrow and I'm not much of a morning person.'

'Shall we have a meal tomorrow after the show then?' I ask.

'That would be lovely,' Julia answers.

Was I asking a young mother on a date or was it Lulu? I don't know, but that's how our relationship began.

16

'Do you know any restaurants that stay open late?' I ask Pat on the Friday morning.

'No such thing,' she says. 'That's why there are so many private members' clubs. Why do you ask?'

'Oh, I'm just going to a play and thought I'd eat after rather than before,' I lied. I didn't want to tell her I was going on a date with a client.

'Well, that's not a problem then. The salt beef bars in Soho stay open until midnight.'

'The play's on at the Royal Court,' I say, then bite my lip. I'd given her too much information.

'Brucie, that's very brave of you. What if Miss Foster sees you in the audience? No! You *want* her to see you in the audience. Why don't you just be a brave boy and ask her out? I'm sure I know what her answer will be.'

I couldn't hide the truth.

'Okay, so we're getting together after the show. But everything's closed by then around here. Where can we go?'

'Ask Mr Singleton. Just don't tell him you're dating a client. And by the way, have you seen that picture of Miss Foster outside the theatre, and how many men in trench coats gather around it?'

Pat's eyes danced with mischievous delight.

'And just to bring your feet back to terra firma, Mrs Wax rang this morning. Trixie's temperature dropped a degree yesterday and she says Trixie will give birth today. If that happens, Mr Singleton says he will do the lunchtime ops and you can do a home visit.'

In 1971 obesity was only just starting to be a problem in dogs. That morning Boris, an overweight seven-year-old Pug, was carried by his owner, Margaret Carruthers, up the stairs to my consulting room. When she placed Boris on the floor he quickly walked behind her and I could see he was lame on his right hind leg. My appointment sheet had already given me that clue. Brenda had written 'lame' as the reason for Boris's visit.

'When did he first go lame?' I ask.

Running up the stairs yesterday afternoon,' Mrs Carruthers tells me. 'He didn't yelp or anything, but when he got to the top of the stairs he was limping. It hasn't got any better. I have felt everywhere and he doesn't seem to be in pain, but he's still holding up his leg.'

Basil had torn a knee ligament, the anterior cruciate ligament. I need to examine him to eliminate other causes of his lameness, but Mrs Carruthers had told me when the injury happened and how Boris behaved afterwards. I had already looked at Boris and seen he was fat and not bearing weight on a hind leg.

I lifted him onto the examination table, found no swellings or heat in any of his joints, nor pain when I flexed the joints, but felt a looseness, a laxity in the knee joint when I pushed the lower bone, the tibia, forward while holding the upper bone, the femur, in place.

'He's torn a knee ligament,' I explain, and Mrs Carruthers praises the veterinary profession's unique and outstanding abilities to make a diagnosis without the patient's owner saying what's wrong. Now I love the praise, but why is it that perfectly sensible people, often parents who have taken their own children to their doctor, forget that what vets do is pretty much the same as what paediatricians or emergency and critical care medics do – listen to why the patient is there, observe their patient's behaviour, examine and treat?

'Mrs Carruthers, Mr Singleton will repair Boris's torn cruciate but first we have to get some weight off of him.'

Back in those days I felt that all torn cruciate ligaments needed to be surgically repaired. Today, I know I don't have to put small dogs like Boris through surgery, that all I need do is get his weight back to normal, and connective tissue repair in the joint will be just about as effective and as pain free as surgery. Large dogs do need surgical repairs, but the risk of torn cruciates can be reduced in the first instance by keeping a dog's weight under control. The most common way dogs tear their cruciates is landing heavily after jumping for a ball. The sure-fire way to ensure dogs jump high then land heavily is to throw the ball with a tennis-ball thrower. These items are the bread and butter of orthopods.

Mrs Carruthers turns to Boris. 'You must lose weight, so don't eat everything I give you,' she says.

'Do you think he's listening?' I ask.

Boris was sitting quietly on the floor, looking up at his owner. I knew from the expectant look on his face that he was anticipating a food treat, and sure enough Mrs Carruthers takes out a small tin from her handbag, unscrews it and gives Boris a little piece of chicken.

'He knows my threats are empty ones,' she says, and I don't know whether she is being droll or living in a different constellation.

'We really have to get his weight down!' I tell her. 'Otherwise Mr Singleton won't operate. Surgery won't be successful if Boris continues to put more strain on the ligament than it was built to handle.'

'Yes, I understand,' she says. 'But he's very demanding. What do you suggest?'

'Whatever you're feeding him, cut it back by 10 per cent today and another 10 per cent in ten days.'

'But he'll think I'm starving him,' Mrs Carruthers replies, with concern in her voice.

'Not if you do it that way, a little at a time. You can still give him treats but 10 per cent fewer treats. He won't notice. There's another alternative. Pedigree has a low-calorie tinned food called Obesity Diet. It's tasty and filling but low in calories. We can feed him that.'

'Something called Obesity Diet? Certainly not! He's not obese!'

'So you'll reduce his food then?' I ask, and Mrs Carruthers finally agrees.

Trixie had gone into labour at 9 am and had not produced any pups by 11 am, so Brian took over my remaining appointments and I hailed a taxi to Mrs Wax's enchanting Regency home on Acacia Road in St John's Wood.

Topiary. That figures, I thought, as I walked through the front garden and rang her doorbell.

Mrs Wax's Irish housekeeper meets me at the door and takes me to the kitchen, where Mrs Wax is with Trixie, who is lying quietly in a wooden whelping box.

'Her contractions have weakened and I can't feel a pup in the birth canal,' she says to me as a hello.

'Hello, Trixie,' I say, sit down beside her and turn to Mrs Wax.

'When did her waters burst?' I ask, and am told two hours previously.

'And you've had a feel inside and can't feel anything?'

Mrs Wax confirms that is correct.

'Do you mind if I have a feel?' I ask, and when she answers in the affirmative I wash my hands in Betadine, put some KY jelly on my baby finger and feel inside. Curiously, it isn't until years later that I start to use gloves for these exams, for emptying anal sacs, even for surgery. We didn't worry anywhere near as much as we should have about infection.

I can't feel anything either and tell Mrs Wax I'd like to give an injection to induce more contractions, and as she has no objections that's what I do. Soon Trixie is pressing down once more with wonderful, full contractions, but I can still feel nothing in the birth canal and can see tension in Trixie's eyes. It is hurting and frightening her.

'Mrs Wax, either the first pup is a breech or its head is too large to pass through the pelvis, but I'm afraid Trixie needs a caesarean and as soon as possible.'

'I thought that was the case,' she replies. I telephone the surgery to get prepared for the op.

'Take the whelping box,' Mrs Wax tells me. 'I want her to wake up in it.'

I put it in the back of her cream Volvo estate, then with Trixie on my lap Mrs Wax drives us to Pont Street, where I take her downstairs for Brian to do an immediate caesarean section.

Brian and Pat are waiting, and Brian has wheeled out the old ether anaesthetic machine.

'Have you performed a c-section before?' Brian asks. As a student I had done one of most operations, opening stomachs, intestines or bladders, removing spleens, kidneys or lobes of lung, but I'd never done a caesarean. In fact, I hadn't seen a gravid uterus, a uterus filled with the about to be born, since I did experimental surgery on pregnant sows two years previously.

'No, I haven't,' I answer.

'Then this is a good opportunity,' he says. 'The trick is in the anaesthetic and the speed of your removal of the pups from the uterus. The longer you take, the more anaesthetised they become. That's the reason for high mortality in caesars. With a small litter, you should have all the pups out within three to four minutes of her being anaesthetised.'

'If you're operating, I'd prefer to use halothane,' I explain.

'Yes, indeed,' Brian replies. 'As you'll be operating and I'll be the anaesthetist, for a c-section I prefer to use what I know best.'

In retrospect, that was a powerful early lesson for me. If in your hands a treatment is safe and it works, think carefully about changing to a new treatment just because it's new. Brian is now using halothane but still feels more comfortable with ether. In the same way, I used halothane for the next fifteen years before I moved on to the next generation of inhalant anaesthetic, isoflurane.

'Bruce, what have you given her?' Brian asks, and I tell him only oxytocin to induce contractions.

'Good,' he replies. 'The fewer injectables the better. We'll mask her down with ether. I use atropine to control salivation and pethidine to make masking down easier. He injects Trixie with both.

Ten minutes later, as I scrub up for surgery, Brian lifts Trixie's forelimbs so that she stands on her hind legs, and Pat shaves her belly and gives it a scrub with Betadine. Then Brian wraps Trixie under his arm and puts the ether mask over her face. The smell of ether where I am standing six feet away is dramatic and I wonder who will be asleep first, Brian or Trixie, but she succumbs quickly, and is intubated and on her back with her legs tied in position within seconds. Pat, who has already opened the surgical towels and instrument pack, gives Trixie's belly a final cleanse with surgical spirit and I prepare to operate.

'Bruce, a good, long incision. Four inches. Just clamp and leave the skin bleeders.'

I do so.

'Same length along the linea alba.* Small scalpel incision at the anterior end, then use the scissors. The uterus is flush against the linea alba and you don't want any accidents,' Brian explains.

I cut into Trixie's abdominal cavity and her turgid uterus fills the site.

There's always melodrama in surgery. The fiery reds, the inherent beauty of vital organs. A caesarean is the most melodramatic because all the tissues are vital and healthy looking and inside are perfect living beings. There's no purple or black as there is if a peach stone has ground to a halt and destroyed the blood supply to a section of intestine. There's no deeply evil-looking change to normality that cancers cause. Caesareans are theatrical and, when all pups survive, the most satisfying of all operations.

'Now a longitudinal three-inch incision by the neck of the uterus over the first pup. That one is most at risk, so get it out fast and hand it to Pat.'

I incise the uterus, squeeze the pup back until its head is in the incision site, then, 'milking' it from its tail end, squeeze it and its afterbirth out and hand it all to Pat, who wipes mucus from its face, shakes it down a couple of times, clamps and cuts the cord, then vigorously rubs it with the warmed towel in her hands.

'All hands on deck!' Pat shouts in the direction of the stairs.

---

* The symmetrical abdominal muscles on both sides of the body meet in the middle. Dogs and cats have vestigial belly buttons, so this meeting line is very distinct and called the 'linea alba' or 'white line'.

'Bruce, faster,' Brian gently admonishes, and I milk out the next pup from the same horn of the uterus, hand it to Brian, then another from the other horn, handing it to Brenda, who has responded to Pat's call.

'This one's a bruiser,' Pat says as the first pup lets out a squeal. 'I remember my first caesarean,' she continues, as she swaps pups with Brenda and vigorously rubs the third pup's body with one of the towels that has been warmed in the dog wash drying cupboard. I am tense with worry that Brian is watching me operate and the pups might not survive and Pat's mind is back at the beginning of time.

'Was that with me?' Brian asks.

'Oh, no, Mr Singleton. Long before you. It was when I was doing farm work with Mr Fennel. Mr Fennel had stripped to the waist to do what he thought would be a difficult but normal delivery but couldn't reposition the legs and he asked me, because his hands were huge and my hands are small, if I could use my fingers to try to push the calf's knee back.'

I pull out a fourth pup and hand it to Brian.

Pat continues, '"You're letting *her* do it?" the farmer asked and Mr Fennel told him he was, and the farmer said. "Does she strip to the waist?" I thought it was very funny, but Mr Fennel was very affronted and told the farmer in no uncertain terms to leave the barn at once and not come back until he was finished.'

'Get your fingers in,' Brian tells me. 'Are there any more?'

There is. A fifth and final pup in the most distant part of the uterus near the ovary. I milk it down to the incision site, squeeze it and its placenta out, and hand it to Pat.

'Bruce, well done. Just under seven minutes. You'll be faster next time,' Brian says, and I take that as a great compliment from a man who doesn't freely give them.

'That's the excitement over. Now it's a simple and mundane closure. You can see how the uterus is already contracting. Place a continuous line in the myometrium, then invert it with another line, then close the visceral surface with mattress sutures. Mrs Wax will want more pups from this dog. I'll leave you to it,' and Brian leaves.

I sew up Trixie's uterus, then do a routine closure of her abdomen, placing the skin stitches under her skin so there will be no sutures the pups might try to suckle from. When I finish, I put Trixie in her whelping box where the RANAs have already put the five pups and two hot water bottles covered in sheep fleece.

Brenda pushes each pup's head into a teat and each pup latches to its mother.

'I'll sit with her until Mrs Wax comes,' Brenda says. 'It must be so strange feeling uncomfortable, falling asleep, then waking up feeling really uncomfortable with all these "things" around.'

I've never thought of my patients that way: what it's like to be a dog, what they think about, even if they think at all.

'Darn. I forgot to ask Mr Singleton about restaurants,' I mutter to Pat, as she clears away the mess in the operating room.

'No worry. I asked,' Pat replies. 'He says the Intercontinental Hotel restaurant at Hyde Park Corner is the nearest and serves until midnight.'

I didn't think my stomach would last until 11 pm for dinner, so back upstairs I made myself a cheese omelette and later telephoned Mrs Wax to see how Trixie and her pups were. At 10 pm, I was at the Royal Court stage door with more freesias, and this time Julia's dressing room was empty of visitors when I arrived. She was in the same body-clinging satin dressing gown. It had a good body to cling to.

'Oh, it was so embarrassing last night,' she says as she kisses me hello. *She kissed me hello!* I hand her the freesias.

'You must think we're all terribly vain and theatrical, but it isn't always like last night. It's just that Oscar wanted me to meet Joel, and Frank has just finished a play he's written for me, and, well, I'm so sorry you got caught up in all of that. Now, you must be famished.'

'I thought we might get something to eat at the Intercontinental,' I say.

'Wonderful. It will only take me a few minutes to change,' Julia replies.

'I'll wait out in the corridor.'

'That's okay,' she says. 'Just turn around,' which I do, and a few minutes later we are in her red Mini, talking about the play, heading for Hyde Park Corner. I learn the play is moving in a week to the Apollo Theatre on Shaftesbury Avenue and she has been nominated for Actress of the Year in the *Evening Standard* Theatre Awards. There is no place to park by the hotel, so Julia parks her car on the pavement. I try to open the door to the restaurant for her, but she gets there first.

We both order club sandwiches and I ask her what other plays she has done. 'My most recent was a David Mercer play with darling Michael Hordern. It was called *Flint*.'

'You were in that? I saw it,' I explain.

'What did you think of the play?' she asks, and I tell her I thought she was wonderful in it.

'Yes, but what did you think of the play?' she repeats, and I realise that it must have been a trite story because although the acting was crystal clear in my mind, the plot had already become fuzzy.

'Last night you mentioned to Joel Grey that you've acted with a "Tommy" and Anthony Newley. Was that in plays?'

'That was in films, *Half a Sixpence* with Tommy Steele and *The Small World of Sammy Lee* with Anthony Newley.'

'Wow. You've done films.' I don't know what else to say.

'Oh, yes. I was Gilda, the girl that Michael Caine gets pregnant in *Alfie*. I was Jonathan Miller's sister in *One Way Pendulum* and went to bed with Oliver Reed in *The System*.

'So I should know you,' I respond, and she giggles.

'How did you become an actress?'

'Well, that's a long story, but let's just say I wasn't very good at school but discovered that I could be very good at pretending to be someone else when on stage or on camera. But more importantly, how did you become a vet?'

I explained that in my family it had always been assumed I'd study human medicine, but I had a little rebellion and shifted to veterinary medicine when I learned that my best buddy, whom I had travelled around Europe with six years previously, was going to do so.

'Have you always had dogs?' I ask, and I learn about Andy, a nippy fox terrier and Wickham, her parents' present Beagle.

'And Honey?' I ask. 'She's a beautiful dog. I've never lived with a dog her size. What's it like?'

She leans forward, smiling. 'Like having a second nanny.'

'You have a *first* nanny?' I ask, and Julia tells me about Rita, her daughter's nanny, and Jim, Rita's husband, who also lives with them.

'My parents live in Brighton,' she continues. 'I couldn't work as I do without a nanny.'

'So, a daughter, a dog, a nanny, a nanny's husband and a busy career. I guess there's not much time for socialising.' I am feeling my way through to asking her out on another date.

'No, there isn't,' she giggles. 'I have a matinee and evening performance on Saturdays, and I'm exhausted on Sundays. Of course, Rita has Sundays off.'

'I could walk Honey for you,' I suggest. 'She's the size of dog a guy's happy to be seen in public with.'

'Oh, that's so kind of you. Jim, Rita's husband, just adores taking Honey to Kensington Gardens on Sundays.'

'While he's doing that maybe you and Emily and I can do something. We can go to a movie,' I suggest, and Julia radiates a smile. I'd noticed that Walt Disney's *Fantasia* was on at a cinema in Soho, thought that might be interesting to a child and suggest we go there. Julia agrees. We have a date.

Years later, I asked Julia what she had thought about when I suggested that the three of us get together for a first date. She told me she thought to herself that almost all the people she knew – mostly actors, producers and directors – were self-centred egoists interested only in themselves. I was different, unworldly, quiet, looked after the welfare of animals, so I must be a good guy, that I was the type of man you marry.

I can see how she came to that conclusion, but I still don't know why I suggested that her three-year-old join us on our first date. It may well be that I was the type of person a woman should marry. Equally, it may be that I'd do anything to get her into my bed.

17

Just after dawn broke I went for a ride on Euripides. Julia, Emily and I had our first date that Sunday afternoon, but mid-morning I drove the Morris Minor estate to Mrs Wax's and docked her pups' tails. That's what we did then. Trixie was surprisingly comfortable, considering the major surgery she'd had. There was a little inflammation to her incision but the cut itself was hidden in a fold of tissue caused by her enormous milk production. She contentedly allowed all her pups to nuzzle and suckle, and I marvelled, as I would years later when my own children were born by caesarean section, at how a mother's instinctive rewards from caring for her newborn can overcome the pain of major surgery.

Mrs Wax was exacting about the length of tail she wanted the pups to retain, showing me precisely where she wanted them cut. Their tails were so small I could feel with my fingers where the nearest space between two bones was, then squeeze hard with my nails to crush through that space and rotate each tail off. Trixie looked worried when each pup squealed, and thoroughly licked each one when I returned them to her. I asked Mrs Wax if she wanted me to remove their dewclaws* at the same time, and she told me this wasn't necessary.

---

* Dewclaws are the claws on the digits on the inner sides of the forepaws.

My date with Julia, if it could be called that, was a non-event. I felt like a loose end. She tried to talk to me but concentrated on Emily's demands. They were constant.

'Oh dear,' she murmured when I drove her home. 'We didn't really have a chance to talk, did we? Never mind.' And she put her hands around my waist, pulled me to her and gave me a kiss on my lips. I brightened up, and we made a date to get together again, next time without Emily.

Julia might have thought that I was the type of person you marry, but in the spring of 1971 I still didn't think much at all about the future. I certainly had no idea that two years later we would tie the knot, with Emily our flower girl. I wasn't yet a planner. My high school principal was right. I coasted. Never pushed myself. Relied on luck. And throughout life, good luck has been and continues to be on my side. I think I know why.

By nature I'm an optimist. That's simply the way I was born, and from what I've read that puts me in a minority, a fortunate minority. How do people – parents – respond to a happy baby? Of course we smile more at them. We pay more attention to them. If you hand out rewards, you get them in return. My parents might deny it, but they paid more attention to me, they 'nurtured' me more than my older brother, who I could say was born genetically neutral, neither an optimist nor a pessimist.

I was born with an array of genes that expressed themselves in a way that made me a natural optimist, but I was also born with a vast number of other genes, you could call them 'pessimist' genes that were 'quiet', not activated. The way I was nurtured suppressed those genes. They never expressed themselves. On the other hand, my 'optimist' genes were nurtured even more. Geneticists now understand that the influence of nurture is so profound it means the way I was raised not only influences my adult personality, in turn it has influenced the genetic make-up of my own children.

Psychologists also understand the direct link between the 'optimist' personality and the ability you have to give your 'cool' emotions control over your 'hot' ones. When I was little, intuitively, I saved the best part of my meal for the last. I didn't go for the instant reward, I postponed it. I didn't train myself, at least not at first and not wittingly, to do so. I just did it.

If you're asking yourself what this has to do with good luck, science has answered that. Those of us either born with the ability to wait for our rewards rather than instantly grab them, or who learn how to do so, do better in exams, have more successful marriages, are healthier, are more content and live longer. We are even thinner!

In 1971 I was also discovering that my inherent optimist's approach to discussing medical conditions with pet owners reassured them. They were grateful to hear good news as well as what was often bad news. With a fractured bone, for example, my inclination to lead with the positive, to say, 'In six weeks he'll be fit as a fiddle, and for that to happen we need to put a metal pin in the bone then make sure he rests his leg and doesn't act like a jerk,' resulted in people asking to come back to specifically see me. Even when the news was dreadful, my inclination to say, 'He's very comfortable but ...' or 'Cats are great, they just get on with life but ...' was comforting to pet owners. I'm sure that's why, embarrassingly, so many of Brian's clients found out where I was practising after I left his employment in early 1973.

Julia and I continued to see each other occasionally in the following weeks for late meals after she came off stage. Mery came down from Cambridge for a weekend, and we discussed whether he should go into agricultural or companion animal practice after graduating. I was starting to question what I was doing at Brian's. Was it frivolous, looking after people's pets? My clients would visit their hairdressers, then visit me. Both of us served our customers' special needs but we talked about whether either was really necessary. We had no difficulty agreeing that agricultural animals had a utility, had a purpose, but dogs and cats? Would the world be any different without them? Mery concluded that after graduation he would join a mixed agricultural and companion animal practice to discover where he felt most comfortable.

Miss Williams successfully raised the three orphan kittens the dustmen had found, and when they were eight weeks old they moved on to their permanent home with Mick Bullock and his wife. Brian agreed that we would spay them free of charge as long as this didn't interfere with other ops, and Brenda arranged that Miss Williams bring these cats and four more that she had rescued to the surgery one Saturday after we had finished our morning appointments. Brenda offered her afternoon to help me with the operations.

'Dr Fogle. Thank you. Thank you,' Miss Williams repeats after she carries seven cat carriers into the waiting room from the minicab she has hired to transport them.

'For you. For you,' she says, and she hands me two brown and white porcelain figurines of spaniels.

'Gosh. Thanks. But what's this for?' I ask.

'I saw you liked them when you visited,' she replies. She is right. I had noticed them on her mantelpiece when I visited with Brenda, although I hadn't asked about them or touched them. Miss Williams's nervous demeanour reminds me of a hungry ferret, but I now know she isn't as vacant as I thought.

'There's really no need,' I start to say, but she interrupts me.

'Doulton. They're Doulton,' she says, and I know I shouldn't refuse her gift.

While British vets were trained to do flank spays, making the incision on the cat's side, North American vets were trained to do mid-line incisions, making the incision just below the umbilicus on the belly. That's what I did, and Miss Williams watches intently.

'Very good. Very good. That's very good. Looks much better,' she comments.

She liked the fact that the shaved area on the belly was not visible after surgery, as it was on flank-spayed cats. I had seen how the shaved hair on flank-operated cats sometimes grew back a slightly different colour, especially on Siamese and Burmese, and wondered why the UK vet schools taught the flank technique. I still don't have a good answer for that for pet cats, although for feral cats in neuter and release programmes the risks of post-op complications once the cat is back living on its own are less with flank surgery.

One of the cats we operated on that day got very wheezy, and Brenda, who was now more relaxed with me as she could see I wasn't giving up my entire life for an actress, also noticed, as she had before, that a cat's ears got puffy and hot. I wondered whether one of the drugs I was giving these cats was causing this.

To make conversation while I operated, I ask Miss Williams where the other cats have come from and she tells me the University of London. I joke that they must be very academic and she says, 'No. No. V-2s. Bombsites. They live in bombsites. I use these to help them,' and from her shoulder bag she pulls out a massive wire-cutter.

I stop and stare. 'What do you use that for?' I ask, and this tiny canary of a woman explains that she uses the wire-cutters to sever the chain-link fence that surrounds World War II bombsites so that she can provide fresh coley fish from Selfridges food halls for the feral cats.

'There are more. British Museum. More cats. Can you do them?' she asks. I look at Brenda, who turns to Miss Williams.

'Yes, of course we can. If you catch them, we will sterilise them,' Brenda says.

'When you catch them, may I come along?' I ask, and Miss Williams nods her head like a nodding donkey.

'It takes time,' she says. 'All night.'

It was on a Friday evening, well, Saturday morning to be more precise, that Julia's and my relationship became truly personal. The previous 24 hours were quite shocking. On Thursday evening, Frank had invited me over to his place for a drink. I knew he wanted to talk to me about my working for him, but when I arrived at his New Kings Road surgery he was more serious that I had seen him, more perplexed.

He gave me a wry smile when I arrived and a warm hug, and with his arm still around my shoulder we walked through his waiting room into his examination room and then upstairs, where he poured whiskies for both of us.

'Bruce,' he says. 'You never know. You just never fucking know.'

I stay silent.

'A customer came in this morning – a man I've known for years – and he told me to put down his dogs. I asked why, and he said he just wanted me to do it, and if I didn't do it he would, so I did.'

Frank downs his drink and pours himself another.

'More?' he asks, and I decline.

'His wife died this morning.'

Frank settles back in his chair. 'I didn't know that until the cops arrived at tea-time.'

'She died. I killed his dogs, then he went home and killed himself.'

Frank stares at me.

'You just never fucking know,' he repeats.

I don't know what to say, so I ask what the police wanted, and Frank says they were simply filling in their report, getting the sequence of events in order.

'Why kill yourself?' Frank asks, and all I can say is, 'I don't know.' In my twenties I find it hard to grasp that a person might think life isn't worth living. And I certainly think that suicide is against the natural order of life and that it is against the law, although I have come to realise that the decision to end your life is a personal matter for you and your family to make, and that the state should have no role in prohibiting it.

'Frank, another time,' I say, finish my drink, leave, and find myself fretting more that a couple of innocent dogs had been treated as loose ends and needlessly killed than I think about the man and his wife.

On Friday, Mery joined me at the surgery for the day. I saw Max, the German Shepherd, because he was splashing diarrhoea. His tumour was a benign haemangioma and the incision site had healed perfectly. When he saw me, he wagged exuberantly and leapt up to lick my face. I was happy to see him too. A good-looking German Shepherd is just about as handsome as dogs get, but his behaviour reminded me of what Frank had written about Alsatians in his book *D is for Dog*. 'Like the Germans,' he wryly if racistly wrote, 'they are either at your feet or at your throat.' By the time I started writing books, my editors were so socially correct they changed words like 'urogenital' to 'bottom'.

The rest of the day was pedestrian but for one appointment. Mrs Jacobs and I had known for several weeks that her yellow Labrador, Barney, had liver cancer. When I told her that diagnosis she remained composed, as she had when her husband died of pancreatic cancer six months previously. Brian told me of her husband's death, and I was impressed by how stoically she bore her loss. *Like my dad's family*, I thought. *Stiff upper lip.*

Jaundiced and losing weight, Barney had remained comfortable and retained a good appetite until the day before, when he went off his food and refused to go outside. Mrs Jacobs knew it was time and brought him in for me to put him down. As Mery was there he raised the vein in Barney's forelimb, I injected the concentrated barbiturate,* and Barney quickly and quietly passed away. Mrs Jacobs got on her knees, lifted Barney's heavy, limp head on to her lap and wept.

I was learning that the grief people feel when their pets die can be intense but in most instances people pull themselves together within a few minutes. Mrs Jacobs didn't. Her weeping got louder. Mery knelt down to console her, but she was oblivious to his comforting arm. Her weeping turned to wailing and I too got down to calm her, but to no avail. I excused myself and got Pat. Pat stroked Mrs Jacobs arm but she continued to wail and moan. Eventually, Pat physically raised her up from her dead dog's body, and kneeling together on the floor, Pat squeezed her in the tightest embrace and motioned us with her head to leave the room. I was relieved to do so.

'She was so together when her husband died,' I whisper to Mery, as we stand together outside the door. 'Why is she like this with her dog?'

Mrs Jacobs's wailing became softer and eventually stopped. It seemed to both Mery and me that it took hours, but in fact it was probably less than ten minutes before the door opened and a now composed Mrs Jacobs emerged with Pat.

'I'm so sorry,' she says to me and squeezes my arm hard. 'He was always there for me and now he's gone.'

Mery, along with his girlfriend from Cambridge, Caroline, and I had a snack after work, then went to the Apollo Theatre

---

* Death results from a concentrated overdose of anaesthetic stopping the heart.

to see Julia in *Lulu*. After the play, walking over to Carroll's delicatessen on Windmill Street, we saw a crowd around a street dog that had just been run over by a cab. It was dead. The cabby who had hit it was distraught. Mery and I felt utterly useless. 'I'll take it over to the RSPCA on Jermyn Street,' he said.

Salt beef sandwiches and Cokes lifted us, and Mery questioned Julia about arcane aspects of the theatre and she was delighted to provide him with her very knowledgeable answers. Caroline, a bubbly, effusive and tactile girl joined in. When she spoke to me she grabbed my arm, in case I got away before she finished saying what she wanted to say. They went on to a private members' club they had an invitation to, and Julia drove me back to the surgery on Pont Street, where I invited her in and she stayed the night.

This would have been no more than the natural evolution of our relationship but for a knock on the door early in the morning. Knowing that it might be an emergency, I put on some clothes, raced downstairs and opened the door. It was Rose.

'May I come in?' she asks.

'Rose. Yes. Sure. It's very late. I've got lots of surgery tomorrow. When did you get back?'

Rose comes into the waiting room and sits down on one of the chairs.

'This morning. How are you?' she asks, and she leans forward to kiss me. I peck her on her cheek.

'Fine. Fine. How's your mother?'

'Not good. I'm moving back. Let's go upstairs,' she says.

I didn't know what to do or what to say, so I tell her, 'Maybe not tonight.'

In the low light from the lamppost outside, I can see that she is looking me in my eyes.

'Is there someone upstairs?' she asks, and all I can say is, 'Maybe.'

Rose's head drops, and I feel like the biggest heel in the world. If she is moving back to Boston her mother must be seriously ill, or worse. She wants and needs to be with someone she knows, and Julia is upstairs in my bed.

After a long pause she says, 'It wasn't going anywhere anyways,' gets up, kisses me on my cheek and leaves.

I go back upstairs.

'What was it?' Julia asks.

'An emergency, but I've taken care of it,' I answer.

'Was it bad?'

'Yeah, terrible, but everything will be okay.' At that moment I know that our relationship is going to be different from any other that I have had.

18

By my second summer in London I had learned that I particularly enjoyed eye examinations, although I was still not good with them. Getting my head close to a pet, shining a light into its eye and looking at the rainbow of red blood vessels, the round white end of the optic nerve on the sometimes almost psychedelically yellow and green and blue retina is like looking into the very soul of the animal. When I see shrunken or absent blood vessels, a hereditary condition in some dogs and cats, it's as if I'm looking at a fire that has gone out. I particularly enjoyed treating chronic conjunctivitis by chemically cauterising the inner aspect of dogs' third eyelids. This was done by anaesthetising the dog, turning its third eyelid inside out and dabbing it with a phenol-soaked cotton bud. Then the phenol had to be totally removed, otherwise when the third eyelid flipped back into its normal position the phenol would cause an eye ulcer. We did this probably for the same reason that horse vets line-fired horses' legs, because it was steeped in tradition, not because it worked. It took a few more years before I questioned why I was doing this.

I had also started to learn that illness and injury in pets are seasonal. During spring I had treated several cats injured in falls from upper-floor windows. As sun and warmth returns, so do birds. People open their windows to allow fresh air in and cats, mesmerised by the birds and not quite as agile as their PR suggests, fall out. A one- or two-floor fall is usually inconsequential, often no more than a bumped chin and a little bruising. Falling three or four floors is more serious. Depending on what the cat lands on it splits its hard palate – a result of the force of hitting its chin on the ground being transferred to the roof of the mouth – breaks its jaw, or dislocates or fractures its hip. Falling five to eight floors often kills, but curiously, cats can fall nine or more floors and survive, if they are light in weight. Given enough time in free fall, they become, as it were, flying squirrels and their stretched-out bodies give just enough aerodynamic lift to slow their final descent.

Road traffic accidents in London increased significantly during the summer. Dogs were often let out for the day, even from the expensive, brightly painted homes off the Kings Road. That is how they were treated then. Because traffic was relatively slow, the dog's injuries were often muscular rather than skeletal – nasty bruising from bumps – but there were still fractures, and when Brian took a two-week holiday with his wife and teenage children in August, I had complete responsibility for all surgery, and had a chance to pin bones. I wasn't very proficient. On one occasion, pinning a broken femur in a Great Dane, the only way I could manage to get the two parts of the femur in a straight line was by standing on the operating table and pulling with all my strength on the dog's leg, while Pat pushed the thick, long pin I had already driven up from the fracture site and out at the hip, back down through the fracture into the lower part of the bone. Whenever possible I cast long-bone fractures. Plaster of Paris was messy, but I learned from Brian how to throw a neat cast, cut it lengthwise on both sides just before it became rock hard, then wrap it tightly with elastic bandage. By doing that I could, during the four- to six-week

healing process, give the dog a touch of anaesthetic, open the
cast and check that everything was all right inside.

Infectious disease and fight wounds in dogs also increased in
summer and early autumn, probably because dogs had a greater
chance to meet with each other in warm weather. Fleas were a
considerable problem both to pets and their owners. The flea
powders available at that time were messy and not very effective. And the new flea spray, as Meredith had explained to me,
was an organophosphate nerve gas.

Julia finished her run in *Lulu* during the summer and that
allowed us to have more of a normal life. I took her to the Nag's
Head but also to the Grenadier pub, where she thought that
Tom, the publican, in his white tunic with gold epaulettes, was
far too theatrical. We had dinner with Martin Hensler and John
Gielgud at John's elegant Georgian terraced house on Cowley
Street within earshot of Big Ben, where John and Julia talked
theatre and Martin showed me their aviary at the bottom of
their garden. We met Julia's best friends Frank and Jackie often,
for dinner at their apartment and at their favourite restaurant,
Biaggi's on George Street. Affable and charming Jackie not only
told Frank what he should eat, at Biaggi's she even told *me* what
I should eat. Frank told Julia about a new play he had written,
Notes on a Love Affair, and she told Frank she'd be honoured
to be in it. 'No one writes for women better than Frank does,'
Julia beamed after she learned of that play. Between the friends
I'd made, Julia's friends and the local vets, I was feeling comfortable in London. It was getting to be a good fit. I was even
unwittingly starting to sound British. When one morning someone asked how I was, I was shocked to hear myself say, 'Can't
complain.'

Annabelle was given one of her two weeks of holiday in late
August and I was surprised by how much I missed having her
at the surgery. She had a natural affinity with dogs. She could

calm even the most worried shepherd or pointer. Annabelle had been annoyed with me after I docked Mrs Wax's pups' tails.

'The Welsh puppy farmers do it because they know people want to buy puppies that look like they do in dog shows. But why didn't you convince Mrs Wax to leave her puppies tails alone?' she asked.

I really hadn't thought about it. If people asked me to dock tails, I docked tails.

'Would you crop ears too?' she asked, and I told her I knew how to do it but because it wasn't done in Britain I wouldn't.

'You wouldn't because we don't do it here or you wouldn't because it's not fair on dogs to do it to them?' she countered.

She had a point. I knew it was uncomfortable for Dobermans, Schnauzers, Great Danes and other pups when at four to five months of age they had half of their ear flaps surgically cut off because people thought they looked better with erect, pointed ears. When Annabelle forced me to think about it, I realised I was happy that this was a forgotten tradition in Britain because it meant I didn't have to put dogs through a pointless and unpleasant operation. But I wasn't yet generalising my concerns about the welfare of my patients. Eventually I would, made to think by people like Annabelle.

19

I had seen my parents only once in over a year. During the late summer of 1971 they visited for a few days on their way to a holiday in the Austrian Alps. The government had just sold off Thomas Cook, the travel agents it owned, and I got a great travel package for my parents. They met Julia briefly for a pub lunch at the Grenadier. They also met Brian and his wife Hilda, saw where I lived and where I worked. I did speak with my mother frequently on the phone. Twice a month I would phone the overseas operator and ask her to make a person-to-person call to Bruce Fogle, my mother would answer the phone, say he wasn't there, then call me back at the cheaper station-to-station rate. We wrote to each other often. Growing up, when I looked in my father's eyes I didn't see me. When I listened to him, I didn't hear my voice. We were not peas from the same pod. We never had a single interesting conversation. I felt closer to my uncles than to my father, but now, with his writing rather than speaking, I discovered that he had a mind of his own and, unexpectedly, a sense of humour. I started to get to know him.

When Julia was not working, we visited her parents on most weekends at their home just north of Brighton.

'Has anyone ever told you your father looks just like Trevor Howard?' I say to Julia after I first met Dick, an estate agent, and Julia just rolls her eyes. I wasn't the first person to say that. Jean, Julia's mother, small and naturally blonde like Julia, always neat, always dressed with a northern European primness, prepared traditional Sunday lunches, a chicken or joint of meat, dark gravy and overcooked vegetables. It was like Friday night dinner with my family. Julia's grandmother Matt lived with her parents. I was amused when I saw her late one evening alone in the living room, standing to attention when television transmission ended for the day and the BBC played 'God Save the Queen'. With a patriotic grandmother and an equestrian-loving, 'war hero' father – as well as looking like a moustachioed Trevor Howard in an action film, Dick had been evacuated from Dunkirk – Julia's family was cartoon British but also warm and loving. They made me miss my family, and I arranged with Brian that I would have my two weeks' holiday at Christmas time and fly to Toronto. I didn't tell my parents until December that Julia would join me.

Home visits continued to be one of the best parts of working in London, and in the autumn home visits got more exciting. Touring circuses – Billy Smart's, Chipperfield's, Hoffman's – visited Shepherd's Bush Green, the Oval in Kennington and other London locations. London vets had learned that I'd worked at Regent's Park Zoo, contacted Brian and I went on 'home visits' outside our Knightsbridge, Victoria and Chelsea catchment area, sometimes as far as Croydon, to see zoo animals with problems. I wasn't much good.

At Chipperfield's Circus I lost my thermometer up young Camella's backside while taking that elephant's temperature. I was called to the Oval to see a tiger with what her keeper called 'tiger disease' – vomiting and very smelly diarrhoea. I took a stool sample for Jean Shanks's lab to culture (all they found were *E. coli* and Clostridial bacteria, the type of microorganisms you'd expect to find in diarrhoea poop) and couldn't think of anything else to do but treat her with antibiotics. When I asked the keeper why he called it 'tiger disease', he explained that it was the most common problem tigers got.

Billy Smart's Circus was making what proved to be its last seasonal visit to Shepherd's Bush Green, although I would have contact with them again a few years later, when Biba, a trend-setting fashion store on Kensington High Street, asked me to look at penguins, rented from Billy Smart's, living in their roof garden. These Antarctic birds had 'bumble foot', an infection caused by standing in muddy water, and my treatment was to send them back to Billy Smart's. (The Biba roof garden flamingos stayed.)

I visited Billy Smart's Circus to see one of their elephants with a discharging facial abscess. I had a 100 ml bottle of 'procaine and benzathine penicillin' with me but had no idea how much to give an elephant. Fortunately, Malcolm Hime was at the zoo when I called him from a local telephone box, and he told me to give a full bottle every three days until the abscess healed. By the time the touring circus moved on, the abscess looked as if it had healed, although knowing as I do now that the source of the abscess was probably a tooth root, I wouldn't be surprised if the abscess returned once I lost contact with the elephant. What was reinforced was how useful it was, and still is, to have ready access to people who know a lot more than I do.

Circus animals worried me more than zoo animals. I thought it was degrading, seeing these beautiful wild animals – black bears, panthers, monkeys, lions, in their Victorian iron cages or tethered by leg chains – captive for our pleasure alone, not for their own well-being or for enhancing knowledge. But I never saw any abuse of these animals. Not once. If anything, it was the opposite. I saw care and concern from their keepers. I was called at the first sign of illness. Sally Chipperfield's circus Poodles didn't bother me, and I didn't mind if she dressed them for performances. I could see they enjoyed their activities. The performing ponies didn't worry me either. They were domestic animals, bred to work with us. But to see a lion in a cage, listless from infection, or an elephant swaying from side to side in obvious emotional distress, it was horrible. I hated it but, consistent with how I behaved at the time, I did nothing about it.

That autumn I voted for Britain to join the European Economic Community. Before I first came to London I had visited the British Consulate in Toronto with my father's Scottish birth certificate, my parents' marriage certificate and my birth certificate, and had my Canadian passport stamped that I was 'repatriated'. That is why I could vote in UK elections.

Julia had a more exciting vote, as a judge in the *Evening Standard*'s Pub of the Year competition. Twice a week a car picked us up, took us to three pubs, then delivered us home. Julia and I both agreed that the Duke of Cumberland pub on Parsons Green, a four-minute walk from Frank's surgery, was our favourite.

The *Evening Standard*'s car dropped us sometimes at Julia's place, sometimes at the clinic. If I stayed at her place, only Honey knew. I'd leave before Emily, Rita or Jim got up. Honey always walked me to the door, ever hoping I'd take her for a walk, even if the sky was still black. On Tuesdays I had to stay in at Pont Street. I was on call for Frank, Keith, Michael and now John as well. The busiest time was always between 11 pm and midnight. Worries intensify as people get ready for bed and I often had a few emergencies to see. They were usually attended to by 12.30 and the telephone seldom rang again until 6.30 am.

It was a blustery night when the phone rang at 1.30 and Julia, who was staying the night, passed it to me.

'A green python?' Julia hears me say.

'How bad's the burn?' I continue.

'What's it doing now?' I ask.

'So exactly what's the problem?' I reply, then, 'You know how expensive a house visit is at this time of the night?' and 'Okay, it will probably take 20 minutes.'

'What's happened?' a concerned Julia asks.

'Well, it seems that a performing green python at a strip club in Soho bit an electric flex earlier today and burned its mouth. The strippers were concerned about the snake, their boss said he'd get a vet to visit, he didn't, and now the girls have laid down their assets and gone on strike until a vet comes. That's why I can charge what I want.'

'Right then,' Julia says. 'Twenty minutes there. Five minutes to examine the snake. Tell the cabbie to keep his engine running. No peeking, and twenty minutes back. I'm timing you.'

Julia soon started filming a TV series called *Fly on the Wall* for Yorkshire Television in Leeds. We spent weekends together with Honey and Emily in London. I have to say I found Honey more relaxing to spend time with. Emily was a flamboyantly opinionated child. It was and for that matter still is tough to relax with hyperkinetic Emily around. At three years of age, she questioned everything and listened to nothing. I felt more comfortable with Honey, a preternaturally calm individual. The same age as Emily, Honey walked tranquilly by my side, without a lead, when I took her to the park, where she transformed into an agile canine athlete. At Julia's home, Honey was unruffled by visitors, composed when Emily's friends tripped over her, serene in her attitude to the human world that surrounded her. When we visited Julia's parents on weekends and their male Beagle Wickham took a sexual interest in her, she remained self-possessed, disdainful of the lower behaviour of 'dogs', a species she didn't seem to consider herself to be part of. I fell in love with Honey. Julia says I fell in love with her dog before I fell in love with her.

20

In October, I went cat-trapping with Miss Williams at the British Museum. I wasn't too happy when she told me to meet her at her flat at 4 am, but she explained she wanted the cats in their traps for as short a time as possible. We filled the back of the Morris Minor Estate with her traps and a pile of blankets, and drove to the locked front gate of the museum where I parked, and a guard who knew her greeted us and let us in.

'I haven't fed them for two days,' she says to me.

'Very hungry. Very hungry. Don't slam the door. Quiet. Very quiet.'

We unload the traps and blankets.

'You can leave your car there, Sir,' the guard explains.

Silently, Miss Williams carries a wire trap around ten metres to the left, steps over a low wall onto a grassed area, opens the cage, puts some Whiskas rabbit-meat cat food on a piece of newspaper inside it, then trails spoonfuls of the same food in the grass leading to the set trap. She does the same with three other traps in other parts of the grounds, all to the left of the front entrance, and once she is finished we walk over to the main entrance, up the steps and stand behind one of the stone pillars.

'We wait here,' she whispers.

It is only minutes before she hears a trap spring, and when this happens she walks quickly and silently to the trap and covers it with a blanket. I had expected the cats to fight fearsomely when they were trapped, but they remain silent and still. Four cats are in their cages by 6.30 am, and we take them back to Pont Street.

Brenda arrived at 8.30 as planned, we finished their ops by 9.30 and had the cats at Miss Williams's by 10.00. She kept all the neutered cats in her flat until the last remaining unneutered ones had been caught, then released them all. These days, in sterilise and release programmes, cats are returned quickly to where they were caught rather than being housed temporarily elsewhere.

The following Monday was an emotion-laden but inspiring day. The postman arrived, early as always, with a letter from Reverend Foster, whose elderly dog I put down the week before. When Brian first suggested I write letters to families when their pets died, I didn't know what to say, other than to express my sympathy. As the months flowed and I got to know my patients better, it was easier to write because I knew the personalities of the animals I was writing about. Reverend Foster thanked me for my note then continued, 'Many years ago when an adored dog died, a great friend, a Bishop, said to me, "You must always remember that as far as the Bible is concerned, God only threw the humans out of Paradise."'

I'd like to believe in a god or gods, but I don't. By culture I'm Jewish, by religion I'm not. Still, his story was wonderful, and if I've never been able to use it to give me solace when my own dogs died, it has been a balm for some of my clients.

During morning appointments I saw a cat that had fallen from a first-floor window, fortunately with no injuries. After I reassured her owner there was no physical damage, as she was leaving the room she stops, returns and says, 'She didn't fall. My son dropped her out of the window. He wanted to see if she would land on her feet.'

'How old is he?' I ask.

'Twelve,' she replies.

My thoughts go back to when I was twelve years old. Put simply, my friends tortured frogs and snakes. I found what they did repellent, but they remained my friends and I never said anything to any adults.

'Have you discussed his behaviour with him?' I ask and the mother replies she was waiting for my advice before doing so.

My immediate thought is that I am a twenty-seven-year-old single man and she is ten years older and a married parent, so why is she asking for my advice about something that has everything to do with parenting and nothing to do with veterinary diagnostics and treatments? I would learn, a few years later, that she was a 'ticket of admission' client, using her pet to get advice from someone she felt comfortable talking to. She knew her cat had not been injured in its fall but came in nevertheless to ask for my advice about her son's behaviour.

'I would discuss the incident first with your husband, so that both of you send the same message, then with your son, and if it's any consolation, when I was around your son's age I took my cat Blackie up the stairs one day, put her through the railings, cradled her upside down then dropped her. I also wanted to see how fast she righted herself and landed on her feet.'

'Oh god, you have no idea how much better you've made me feel!' she exclaims, clasps my hand and shakes it, and at the same time kisses me.

Other appointments were pedestrian, although I did manage to fish out a sewing needle from a cat's oesophagus. The giveaway was thread hanging from its mouth. His owners had pulled on it at home but it didn't budge. Fortunately, this had not caused any more damage. (Word of advice: If you see thread hanging from either your cat's mouth or anus, don't give anything other than the most gentle pull. The risk of serious damage is enormous.) That cat needed an anaesthetic, so my visit to the Royal Mews to put down an elderly and lame gun dog, already delayed by my taking X-rays of a coughing and feverish Westie's chest, was delayed even more. When I developed the Westie's X-rays I saw a snowstorm in the dog's lungs, phoned the dog's owner and gave her the dreadful news that the lungs were riddled with tumours. She told me she would like her dog put down that day, but would take him home then bring him back at the very end of appointments in the early evening.

The gun dog's owner whom I visited in the Royal Mews was gracious about my delay in getting to him. He had previously asked my advice on the most humane way for him to shoot his dog. I'd explained from the top down rather than from the front towards the back, but had convinced him it would be more humane if I came and did the deed with an overdose of barbiturate, which I did. I had one more visit, simply to vaccinate a German Shepherd at its home on Embankment Gardens. I'd been warned by Pat about Larry Spiegel, this dog's owner. The dog had a penchant for biting strangers' hands, and the owner, for whatever reason, found his dog's behaviour deeply satisfying.

I kept my hands stuffed in my pockets as I walked up the stairs from the front door. Sitting down with the dog's nose intently buried in my pocket, waiting for my hand to emerge, I asked the owner to put his dog's head between his own legs in a knee lock when I vaccinated the big beast. I figured if the dog was going to bite anything, or give an upper thrust with his head, that was the best place for his head to be. I'm sure I'd get sued today if I made a similar suggestion.

Back at the surgery the Westie's owner, a slim woman in her fifties, arrived just after 6 pm wearing a soaking-wet trench coat. The skies, threatening rain all day, had turned charcoal in late afternoon, and cold, stinging rain had descended. Her dark hair stuck to her face, crimson from the sudden chill. Water dripped off her onto the floor around. She was carrying Martha on a red blanket and both were dry.

'Got caught in the rain?' I ask, more to avoid talking about what I am about to do than anything else.

'Yes,' is all she says.

'But Martha's dry,' I say.

'Yes, she is.'

'How's that?' I boringly and insensitively continue.

'When you told me the news,' the woman says, 'and I knew this was the last day of Martha's life, I wanted to take her home and then to Kensington Gardens so that she could have a final visit to her favourite places. But she was too weak to walk, so I put the blanket in the basket of my bicycle so she would be comfortable, then put her in it and took her to the park. I knew it was about to rain so I took an umbrella, and when the heavens opened I was able to keep her dry for her last visit. She adores that park.'

'Can you excuse me for a minute while I get a nurse?' and I leave the room and disintegrate. By now I had put down many pets and was familiar with grief. Yet this woman's simple story of what she has done to make the last hour of her dog's life as pleasing as possible make my shoulders heave. Annabelle finds me in the hallway and intuitively knows why I am bawling my eyes out.

'It's okay. Take a few deep breaths,' she says and I gradually compose myself.

We return to my room, where I give Martha her lethal dose of pentobarb, the normal circumstances reversed, my eyes red with sadness, Martha's owner's clear and sensible. She strokes her dog's head.

'Do you know,' she says, 'that the Eskimos lay the head of a dead dog in a child's grave so that the soul of the dog, which is everywhere at home, can guide the helpless infant to the land of the souls?'

21

Julia finished taping *Fly on the Wall* for Yorkshire Television, and, as planned, we flew to Toronto for her to meet my family on their turf and see where I'd grown up. She met once more my reserved and strikingly handsome father, who was a pushover for any blonde with a good figure. That's what he'd married. My effusive and energetic mother was unenthusiastically warm and gracious to her. Julia met my much younger sister Adeen, going to university, and my older brother Rob and his wife Eileen. Rob worked with our father in the flower shop and Eileen was a school teacher. Just as important to me, Julia met our three Yorkshire terriers, Sparkie, and her daughters Duchess and Misty.

'They're lovely,' Julia comments, 'a bit frenetic, a bit like your mother.'

In Toronto we dropped in on my Fogle aunts, beautiful Mary, frail and petite Jeannie, blousy Edie, prim and observant Nettie, all sensibly dressed in their tweed skirts and laced leather shoes. Julia found them all both familiar and easy. When we met my mother's four surviving brothers, Julia found them more daunting. Bill, the male equivalent of my mother, gregarious, joyous, opinionated, an oral surgeon. Ed, ever thoughtful, ever considerate, articulate, a jazz pianist, a collector of thoughts and words, a lamp manufacturer. Sam, the patriarch, exuberant, jovial, boastful, a hugger, a dreamer. We spent an afternoon with Reub, my favourite, my sounding board, my advisor, a psychiatrist with immense personal demons, a man in need of thoughtful and continuing therapy.

Reub's combined medical office and home was in midtown Toronto. A short man with small facial features he was both a great success and enormous failure. He may have been joking when on graduating from medical school in 1926 he wrote as his motto in the university yearbook, '*When work interferes with pleasure, cut out work*,' but that's how he lived his life. His bloodless tonsillectomy technique, perfected at the Mayo Clinic in Rochester, Minnesota, was front-page news throughout North America in 1929, yet by 1932 he had dropped out of medicine and was road manager to an opera singer he had become infatuated with. 'I knew it wouldn't last when she ate a pastrami sandwich while we made love,' he once told me when I was confiding in him about my girlfriend tribulations.

I had briefed Julia that between then and now he had married and divorced several times, had many nervous breakdowns, had moved from ear, nose and throat to psychiatry, and had recently married Cynthia, a former patient, a foot taller, forty years younger and equally mixed up. In 1962, when I told my family I planned to go to veterinary school, not medical school, and my parents tried to convince me otherwise, it was Reub who defended my corner, who argued with his sister and brother-in-law that it was a noble choice and that I should follow my desires.

'What are your feelings now about veterinary practice?' he asks, and I explain that my greatest worry is whether or not I am making the right diagnoses.

He smiles at Julia. 'It must be very satisfying, being an actress, getting into the thoughts and motives of the characters you play,' to which Julia replies enthusiastically that that is the very reason why she enjoys rehearsals even more than doing paid performances.

Uncle Reub asks Julia about her family, and she explains that Emily and her dog Honey are staying with her parents while we are in Canada. 'Emily can cope with anything, but I do worry a little about Honey,' she says.

'I see many patients who have dogs and I've noted that the affection they feel for their pets is less complicated than the affection they feel for other people, even their children,' says Reub. 'Bruce, do you know that Freud wrote about this? He called the affection we feel for pets *affection without ambivalence*.'

Reub asks me if there is anything I do that has been unexpected, and I tell him I find putting down dogs and cats is the hardest part of work.

'I'm not surprised,' he answers. 'At a stroke you are breaking an attachment that involves deep love. You see the grief that ensues and can't help but feel you have caused it. Do any of your clients get angry with you?' he asks.

'Not when I put down their pets. But sometimes later, when they think I might have been able to do more or didn't make a diagnosis in time or made a wrong diagnosis. That's when some of them get angry with me.'

'Of course they do, even when deep inside they know it's not your fault.'

He got up, went to his bookshelf and brought back a book called *On Death and Dying* by Elisabeth Kübler-Ross.

'This is for you,' he says. 'It was published last year. The author says there are five stages of grief: denial, anger, bargaining, depression and finally acceptance. I'm sure this is what you see in veterinary practice too.'

Reub moves his chair closer to me. I am familiar with this manoeuvre. He lives with my family, often for months at a time after each of his nervous breakdowns. That's how we developed our strong relationship, and I know his mind is racing and he is excited by where it is going.

'I see this all the time,' he continues. 'Breaking an attachment can produce anger and anxiety as well as sorrow. And when I think about it, a pet is a perfect attachment figure. Look at your mother's dog. She's non-threatening. Is that right? Not like your mother.'

All three of us smile at that. I don't know if Uncle Reub added that for Julia or for me, but in either case he was acknowledging that he knew why I was in no hurry to return to Canada.

'You can control your dog,' he continues. 'In fact you control her life completely. She is warm and soft to touch. She's always there in your home. She needs you. She respects you. She thinks you are extra special. Has she ever criticised you or your mother?'

I smile. Julia is feeding off his words.

'Criticism. That's what we hate most. Not constructive criticism. Constant criticism. The constant drip of disparagement. That's why marriages fail. They start with good sex and end with denigration.' He turns to Julia. 'I imagine your dog makes you feel important to him.'

'Yes, she's a she and she does,' Julia replies.

'And you feel she is loyal to you.'

'Absolutely!'

'That you can't think of anyone in the world, other than your parents, who is as loyal to you as your dog is.'

'I've never thought of it that way, but, yes, other than Bruce, I think that's true.'

I butt in on their duologue.

'Uncle Reub, I have a client, a young guy who recently moved from the sticks to London, who got himself a cat for companionship and named her *Mom*.'

'You didn't tell me that,' Julia says turning to me.

'It wasn't something worth telling until now.'

My sister-in-law had organised a meet and greet with her friends and we had to go.

'Uncle Reub, I wish we had more time. And not that you'd be surprised, but you've cracked open a window for me. I've found my patients pretty much as I expected. It's their owners I've had difficulty understanding. I've never really thought about the hidden reasons why they behave the way they do with pets.'

That wasn't exactly true. I had thought about my clients' relationships with their pets, but only in a superficial way. That's why I'd felt I was the equivalent of a hairdresser, making people feel better but in the wider context of life, what I did, other than reducing discomfort for a few dogs and cats, was rather meaningless. My uncle's thoughts got me thinking about why so many people keep pets. Why do so many of us burden ourselves, emotionally and financially, by keeping pets?

After a little more talk, I thanked him for the book and we left. Driving back through the snowy Toronto streetscape to Eileen and Robert's house, Julia, not unexpectedly, says, 'Your Uncle Reub is wonderful! I can't believe he has nervous breakdowns. Can we take him home with us?'

'Every girl wants to take him home,' I answer. 'And no. He's great in small quantities but not 24 hours a day. That's his new wife's job now.'

22

It was bitterly cold, colder than Toronto, when we returned to Britain for New Year's with Julia's parents and their Beagle Wickham, her grandmother Matt, Emily and Honey and Julia's sister Alex. While in Toronto we told my parents we would return in the summer if Julia was free, so that she could visit the cottage on Lake Chemong, the place I considered my true home.

Julia started rehearsals on Frank Marcus's new play *Notes on a Love Affair* and I returned to what had now become the routines of Pont Street. John Rohrbach had sold his Holland Park surgery to Andrew Carmichael, a Cambridge graduate just back from several years at the Animal Medical Center in New York City, and Keith arranged that we'd have lunch together one Saturday. After lunch we returned to Andrew's, where he showed us his 'ultrasound' machine, the first in a veterinary practice in Britain.

'There's a Scot to thank for this,' he pronounces, as Keith and I examine the apparatus. 'Ian Donald in Glasgow,' he continues without our prompting.

'Is that who told you about it?' I ask, and Andrew, whose blond hair cascades down to his shoulders, replies, 'Donald invented it. We used one at the AMC for visualising abdominal organs. I use it for measuring heart activity.'

'Can you do a pregnancy diagnosis with it?' asks Keith, and when Andrew confirms 'yes', we both know we are delighted to have Andrew and his ultrasound machine less than twenty minutes away from both of us. That started the beginning of another close veterinary relationship.

Meanwhile Julia was revelling in rehearsals.

'Robin is the best director I have ever worked for!' she exclaims.

'He told me to think about something Irene says.' Irene is the actress Irene Worth playing a Margaret Drabble-like character, an author named Dora.

'Near the end of the play, Irene says, "Your instinct is more than my imagination." Robin says that says everything about who I am.'

Julia beams with excitement.

'Okay, then. Give me a one-minute resumé of the play,' I ask and Julia replies, 'Well, Frank puts in a little Shaw, a little Brecht, a little Pirandello. Critics might think he's being too European. There's a play within a play. When I first appear, I think life is sort of booby-trapped, but after Irene tricks me into having an affair with her former husband – that's Nigel Davenport – to give her fodder for a play she's writing, I emerge as a poised but pregnant life force.'

'And how would you describe your character?' I ask.

'I'm a timid dental assistant, Jennie. I'm going to dress in all the colours of mouse. I'm shy. I wear glasses. I'm gawky. And I'm completely asexual.'

'Completely asexual?' I ask, and Julia says, 'Yes, I'm not interested in sex. It isn't a priority.'

'And are you going to bring this character home from work the way you did with sexy Lulu?' I ask, but Julia is too excited about rehearsals to hear what I am really saying.

Your instinct is more than my imagination. I thought about that line and it explained why I was so attracted to Julia. Her instinct *was* more than my imagination. She doesn't 'think' the way I do. I mull over stuff, see both sides, am consensual. Julia is instinctive, reactive. And her instincts – about people, about ideas – are more accurate than my thoughtfulness.

A week before Julia is to leave for Southsea, where her play's out-of-town try-out begins, I spay Honey. Meredith and I finish our library research on pain in dogs, and he posts me a simple resumé of what he has read.

- Nociceptors in nerve endings: transmit pain signal through sensory neurons in spinal cord to brain.

Different types of pain:

- Cutaneous – from skin and superficial tissues.
- Somatic – from damaged nerves, blood vessels, ligaments, tendons, bones.
- Visceral – from damaged organs or body cavities.
- Routine spay damages skin, blood vessels and internal organs: ipso facto causes cutaneous, somatic and visceral pain.
- Healthy dog tolerates pain better than sick dog.
- Sick dog less likely to tell you about pain it feels.
- Evolutionary tactic – don't let predators know you're not well.
- Painkillers work better given before pain develops than given later.
- Dogs have identical neurotransmitter chemicals to humans.
- Pain perception occurs in same location in dog's cerebrum as human cerebrum.
- People leave hospital faster, heal, recover, faster when post-surgical pain controlled.

- Pain triggers stress-related hormones. Might explain
  why people given pain control have fewer post-op
  infections than those not given good pain control.

Since Meredith gave me that list there have been great advances
in pain management, but his basis for understanding why pain
should be controlled is as good today as it was then.

I decide to spay Honey on a Wednesday when Brian is doing
elective ops in Surrey. I'll operate at lunchtime, she'll go home
late afternoon, then I'll stay with her at Julia's that evening.
This is fine with Brian. She'll also be my first spay where I
integrate a high level of pain control into her post-op treatment. A half-hour before surgery, I give her ACP, a sedative,
atropine to control saliva, and pethidine, a narcotic painkiller.
She'll get more pethidine four hours later, then continue on
paracetamol and codeine tablets for several days once she is
back home.

I still don't know what triggered Honey's 'anaphylaxis', a
life-threatening allergic reaction. I had already opened her up
and had pulled one horn of her uterus through her incision
when I heard the moistness in her lungs and saw her hanging
lips turn purple.

'Untie her!' I shout to Brenda, who should have been moni-
toring the anaesthetic more carefully, and while she unties
Honey's hind legs I do the same with her front legs. Once this
is done, holding her by her hind legs, I suspend her so that fluid
in her air passages can drain out. Her pink intestines hang out
of the incision in her abdomen like a string of sausages in a
butcher's window.

'Adrenaline!' I shout. Brenda asks how much and I tell her an
ampoule. She draws the liquid into a syringe.

'Intramuscular. Deep. Up here in the thigh,' I direct, and
Brenda gives the life-saving injection.

Honey's breathing gets better as soon as gravity removes the fluid in her air passages. The single injection of adrenaline is sufficient, and once she is stable – only five minutes later – she is tied back on the table and I scrub up once more and complete the spay.

'I'm glad it was a family dog, not someone else's,' Brenda comments.

'*You* might be,' I reply.

Honey's recovery that afternoon was uneventful – no thrashing in the kennel, no crying. When Julia arrived to take her home, the sweet dog walked up the stairs on her own, wagging her tail. She slept in a bed in the hallway, but that evening I moved her bed into Julia's bedroom where all our dogs' beds have remained ever since. Julia, Rita and Jim hovered over her. Emily, who had just celebrated her fourth birthday, made a 'get well soon' card for her with Honey's picture drawn on it.

The following week, with Honey fully recovered, Julia left for Southsea. She'd go straight to Brighton from there, the next town on the play's try-out. On Monday I had a call from Harrods. 'Grimwade here. We have a slight problem. No urgency, but please visit today.' I did, and he invited me into his office.

'One of our special customers has gifted Harrods with her parrot,' he explains. 'She approached the General Manager with her request some time ago, and he accepted. Upon her death we would display her parrot, an African Grey, with signage explaining that we were to find a good home, and the parrot's new owner would make a suitable donation to the Imperial Cancer Research Fund.'

'That's very thoughtful of both Harrods and the bird's owner,' I reply.

'I'd like you to examine the parrot,' Grimwade tells me. I ask where it is, and he explains it has been on the shop floor that morning but for reasons I would soon see has been moved to the pet department's storage room. That's where we go.

The bird is in a sixty-inch-high, thirty-inch-wide brass cage that probably cost the equivalent of four months of my salary. It is magnificent. I walk over to have a close inspection of the bird, and as I move to it, it moves over on its perch to be close to me. It tucks its head down for a top touch once I am beside its cage, and I give it a quick scratch while I examine its droppings on the cage floor then look at the bird itself, watching its breathing, checking the diameter of its 'nostrils', examining the state of its feathers.

'The bird's name is P-O-L-L-Y. Say hello to it,' Grimwade whispers, so I do.

'Hello,' I say, and the bird comes over and asks for another touch.

'No. When you say hello, say her name immediately after,' Grimwade curiously requests.

'Hello, Polly,' I say, following Grimwade's strange request.

Once more the bird waddles along its perch over to me and this time replies, 'Go fuck yourself!'

I look at Grimwade, who tries to remain officious but is failing.

'Say hello once more,' he tells me. I do and the bird says nothing, but when I say, 'Hello, Polly,' the parrot once more responds, 'Go fuck yourself!'

'Is that what you want my advice about?' I ask and he explains it is.

'Well, she's a Congo African Grey, and they're great mimics so she could be profane because she's just copying what she heard around her. But she doesn't swear when you say "Hello," only when you say, "Hello, Polly," so I think she's been trained to do it.

When the bird hears me say 'Hello, Polly' to Grimwade, once more she says, 'Go fuck yourself!'

'So, I think your special customer had an unusual sense of humour and a special place in her heart for Harrods.'

Grimwade tells me he will find a home 'internally' for Polly, from within the management and staff.

There was another coal strike in Britain in January 1972 and another State of Emergency. Flying pickets turned coal and oil boats away from Battersea Power Station and London was enduring rotating power outages. The prime minister, Edward Heath, had just signed the Treaty of Accession for the UK to join the EEC, but the British were more interested in their anachronistic and still immensely irritating class war. I was on call the following night, when I saw one of Frank's clients in the late evening. He'd phoned to tell me his mastiff-type dog had swallowed a roll of ten £20 notes. Jokingly, I asked if we could share the proceeds if I got them out for him, and mirthlessly he replied, 'I don't mind if you slit the bugger from stem to stern. I just want my bloody money back.'

When the dog arrived I pushed a ball of washing soda crystals down its throat and it produced the wad of notes within two minutes. The lights were still on an hour later when one of Keith's clients arrived with her twitching, salivating Scottish terrier. The owner had told me when she rang that her dog had a litter of six three-week-old pups. When I saw the dog, I knew my hunch that she was suffering from eclampsia, a potentially life-threatening lack of calcium, was right. She was in effect sacrificing her life to feed her litter. I had already filled a syringe with 10 per cent calcium gluconate to give intravenously and had my elastic leg tourniquet ready when the lights went out.

When the London Electricity Board turned power off during the strike, it was turned off in entire areas, and only then did I realise there was no torch in the building. I picked up a bottle of alcohol, the calcium gluconate and the tourniquet, went downstairs and drove with the owner in her car to where we could see lights, a few streets away on Beauchamp Place.

'I know Mara in San Lorenzo's,' the dog's owner explained, and we pulled to a halt, went into the restaurant, and within a minute a table was cleared and the now almost convulsing dog was given her slow intravenous injection. Like magic – for that's what calcium is in this situation – the poor dog's muscles relaxed and her tension disappeared. Her mind returned and she licked my hand.

'We're over the crisis but not out of the woods,' I explained. 'The pups need to be weaned off her and she might need more calcium tonight. It's best that I keep her with me but with no lights that's going to be a problem.'

'This might help,' said Mara, the wife of the owner of San Lorenzo's, and she produced a torch, a box of white candles and a steaming bowl of risotto to take back to the surgery.

Julia's play was now running in the West End and her reviews were terrific. At the end of the year, the theatre critics of the *Daily Mail*, *Financial Times*, *Evening Standard*, *New Statesman*, and a new magazine, *Time Out*, all selected her as their Actress of the Year. And, yes, she brought her character Jennie home with her after each performance, but it was the poised life force that Jennie became during the course of each evening, not the asexual brown mouse there at the beginning of each performance.

23

Reading Kübler-Ross's *On Death and Dying* gave me a completely different perspective on what I was observing at the surgery. So too did another book I read a few years later, a non-scientific one called *Anatomy of an Illness as Perceived by the Patient*, by Norman Cousins. In that book, Cousins described how joy and laughter – he loved the Marx Brothers' films – relieved the pain he experienced from his incurable collagen disease.* 'I made the joyous discovery that ten minutes of genuine belly laughter had an anaesthetic effect and would give me at least two hours of pain-free sleep,' he wrote.

I had seen how playing with a ball or being made a fuss of seemed to relieve dogs of some of their chronic pain, but I had also observed that almost every pet owner smiled when they described their pet's antics at home. Pets make people smile. They make us laugh. Think about your own pet in good health.

---

* At that time, 'collagen disease' was used to describe a variety of painful conditions such as rheumatoid arthritis, sclerosis and lupus, in which your immune system turns upon and destroys part of the body. Today it's used more specifically to describe immune-mediated diseases that specifically destroy collagen, a major component of connective tissue.

I'd wager that most of you feel better just thinking about the antics of your dog or cat. I don't doubt that my uncle's comments, together with those two books, led to my interest in the people side of clinical veterinary medicine and to my organising the Human Companion–Animal Bond meeting in 1980, founding Hearing Dogs for Deaf People in 1982, and writing extensively on the relationship we have with the natural world around us.

I had now realised that much of what happens in general practice falls into discrete categories. Trauma affects soft or hard tissue. Infections are mostly viral, bacterial or fungal. Skin gets itchy or inflamed. The gastrointestinal tract gets affected from one end – vomiting – to the other – diarrhoea or constipation. Certain conditions are more common than others, so with familiarity my ability to guess what was happening improved.

After two years of clinical experience, I had carried out around 10,000 clinical examinations and anaesthetised 2,500 dogs and cats and a few birds and turtles. I had completed 1,500 operations and gone on 500 home visits. I was gaining confidence in what I was doing.

At university we learned that Hippocrates, the father of medicine, called on doctors to '*cure sometimes, treat often, comfort always*'. That's what we were taught, to 'cure' animals of their afflictions but now, ever so slowly, it was dawning on me that vets and doctors don't cure their patients. We certainly prevent disease, through vaccination and effective parasite control, but when trauma or illness occur, the patient, be it you or me or our pets, cures itself. I was learning that as a vet, what I was doing was creating better circumstances for the animal to repair itself. I did this by realigning a broken bone, with a pin in the bone or a cast around it, so that it repairs in a straight line. Or giving antibiotics to rid the body of infection to allow the lungs or bladder or eye or whatever was infected to mend itself. I gave painkillers, corticosteroids,* intravenous fluids to overcome clinical shock and restore normal functions – to create a more natural environment for the body to get working again. I was trained to get in and do something. Now, through trial and error, I was learning it was often better to do nothing. That less can be more. When Frank first explained his use of placebos, I was shocked. I thought he used them because he was a poor diagnostician. My experience was now telling me that often there was merit in such benign interventions.

I wasn't the first fresh vet Brian had employed. He was familiar with the novice wanting to do everything then gradually realising that a light touch was often best, and after working for him for two years he was confident that I could manage his practice for an extended period of time in his absence. He accepted a visiting professorship offered to him by Jim Archibald, my surgery professor. Brian told me that in early September he was going to Guelph for three months. Brian, as I've said, wasn't a man to give compliments, but I took it as a great big one that he was leaving his surgery in Pat's and my hands.

Through both clinical experience and attending the monthly meetings of the local veterinary association, I was feeling confident in my ability to diagnose and treat problems in dogs and cats. My Uncle Reub's comments on why the relationships people develop with their pets can be so intense had focused my mind. I felt less judgemental when a pet owner behaved in what I thought was a silly way. In my first year, I hated being called 'uncle'. 'Uncle is going to make you better.'

When I heard that I thought two things: *Get a life!* and *I'm not your dog's uncle!* In subsequent years I would have the

---

* Corticosteroids are 'steroid' anti-inflammatories. Drugs such as ibuprofen are 'non-steroid' anti-inflammatories. Corticosteroids are secreted in the adrenal glands.

opportunity to discuss people's relationships with their pets with psychologists, sociologists and cultural anthropologists, and better understand how comforting it was for the pet's owner to call me, a now twenty-eight-year-old who had grown a beard to try to make myself look older than fourteen, by the term 'uncle'. But even before I got the scientific answers I was far less critical, much more tolerant. When someone would say, 'Look at that fur. Don't you just want to bury your head in it?' I'd now think, 'Yeah, I would.' I didn't mind, as much as I did two years previously, when people talked to their pets the way they talked to other people. I didn't understand exactly why but I was more on their side. The more time I spent with hundreds and hundreds of dogs and cats, the more I realised that each one is a discrete individual, with its own set of thoughts, feelings and emotions, its own personality. A dog or cat's essential behaviours – the need to eat or drink or investigate or mark its territory or have sex – were fixed, but there was a fascinating variation from one animal to another. And I knew absolutely nothing about dog or cat behaviour. We hadn't had a single lecture on that topic at university, and behaviour was never a topic at regional or national veterinary meetings. But a pet's behaviour was a component of almost every examination I did or story I heard.

In late spring, Julia finished *Notes on a Love Affair* and before she started work on an inane film, *All Coppers Are ...* at Pinewood Studios, we visited Paris for a weekend. I had seen a Renoir lithograph, in Harrods, of Renoir's son Claude. It was one of an edition of 950, printed in Paris in 1904. I had bought a Rembrandt etching – now fully paid for with Julia's help – simply because it was a Rembrandt, but I fell in love with Renoir's *Claude Renoir, la tête baissée* and was sure that if a copy were available from Renoir's official gallery on the Left

Bank it would be cheaper than at Harrods. There was one, and it was half the asking price at Harrods.

Julia, still more Lulu than dental assistant Jennie, dressed in suede, sky blue hot pants, long, matching waistcoat and big blonde hair for our flight back to Heathrow, and was mobbed by press photographers on our return. I felt uncomfortable and instinctively backed away. I had done so at previous events when photographers buzzed around her and continued to do the same throughout her acting career. Our children regret my behaviour, for while they have hundreds of press photos of their mother, they have strikingly few pictures of their father, especially during the seven years before I felt confident enough to shave off my beard. Julia had a press clipping service, and these newspaper photos of Julia's return to Britain were duly pasted into clipping albums compiled by her father Dick.

Work continued to be fascinating, and although our treatments were basic compared with today, they were effective. Itchy skin was often treated with calamine lotion. Maggot-infested wounds were cleansed out with bubbling hydrogen peroxide. Pat always invoked her position as head nurse to cleanse these wounds. 'Nothing satisfies me more than seeing the last maggot float off in a sea of pink foam,' she'd tell me, and I'd think, *Nothing? Is the husband you never talk about that boring?*

We saw John Gielgud and Martin Hensler frequently, for dinner at their home or at Drones restaurant, across the street from the veterinary surgery on Pont Street. Drones was suitably theatrical because it was co-owned by the actor David Niven and the lead singer and guitarist with Pink Floyd, David Gilmour. The restaurant produced scrumptious hamburgers. One weekend John, Martin, Julia and I were invited by Julia's wig-maker, Stanley Hall, to his farmhouse in Kent. Emily, now four years old, was invited too, and we travelled there in a London taxi arranged by John.

Julia introduced John and Martin to Emily. 'Emily, this is the distinguished actor Sir John Gielgud and his friend Mr Martin Hensler.'

Emily shakes hands with both and sits herself down between Julia and me.

'Why are you called "Sir"? Are you a teacher?' Emily asks as we start our ninety-minute journey to Kent.

'Oh, no, my dear. Not at all,' John smiles. 'The Queen knighted me.'

'What did she do to you at night?' Emily asks.

'No, she didn't do anything to me at night,' John responds, still smiling. 'The Queen may choose to give a knighthood to any of her subjects. If you receive a knighthood you are entitled to be referred to as "Sir" rather than "Mr".'

'Why did she give you a knighthood and not your friend?' Emily continues.

I see a strained look on Julia's face, but Martin is enjoying the exchange.

'You see, the Queen felt I am worthy of one but Martin is not.'

Martin corpses with laughter.

'What I mean is the Queen had seen several plays I was in and felt that I was worthy of a knighthood.'

'My Mummy is in plays. Will the Queen give her a knighthood?' Emily asks.

'For a lady, the Queen bestows a damehood rather than a knighthood, and yes, when she's older the Queen might make your mother a Dame,' John replies.

'Are you married? Where are your children?' Emily continues. She is now bored by talk about knighthoods and damehoods but never tires – still doesn't – of asking questions. Until she is in her twenties, Emily's brain rarely slows down long enough to listen to any answers.

'No, I'm not married and I don't have children,' John replies.

'Why not?' Emily continues, but Julia intervenes before what Martin and I both think would be an exciting answer.

At Stanley Hall's I knew exactly where not to sit. I had met Stanley through his parrots at Pont Street and at lunch he set a table for his ten guests, each of whom had a parrot on a perch behind their chair. One of them, Ethelred the Ready, a blue-fronted Amazon, whose nails I had clipped at the surgery, was a notorious nipper. Stanley thought it immensely funny when, during lunch, Ethelred would silently lean forward and nip the ear of the unsuspecting guest.

John and Martin decided to stay on at Stanley's, and Julia was certain it was to avoid another ninety minutes locked in a vehicle with an inquisitive four-year-old, and we had their taxi take us back home to Julia's. After she puts Emily to bed and we sit down on the sofa, she cuddles up and says, 'Let me show you how clever Honey is,' and calls her dog over.

'Honeybun. Take off my ring,' she says, and obediently Honey puts her mouth around Julia's finger and starts to gently work at removing the ring from it. She wags intently. Honey obviously loves doing this, and after no more than a minute of licking and gently pulling with her incisors, she removes Julia's ring from her finger and marches around the room, as proud as a performing Tennessee Walking Horse.

'Brilliant dog!' I say, and gave Hun a big pat on her back.

'Where's my ring?!' Julia cries out. When I thumped Honey with a congratulatory pat, she accidentally swallowed it.

'What are you going to do?' a grim-looking Julia sternly asks.

'We've got two choices,' I reply. 'Let nature take its course and wait until it comes out the other end, or I can give her something to make her bring it up.'

'I'm not waiting for two days,' Julia says, and I borrow her car, go to Pont Street, get a vial of apomorphine,* bring it back and, a minute after I inject it, Julia's ring is returned to her.

'Don't you ever do that again,' she tells me. I don't know whether she means saying yes to watching Honey's party trick, giving her dog an enthusiastic thump or making the innocent creature vomit, so I just give an affirming nod.

---

* Apomorphine, a drug that induces vomiting (and has nothing to do with morphine).

24

I may be a natural optimist but that doesn't mean life always goes as planned. It is an unexpectedly hot and radiantly sunny June morning. Hyde Park is a mosaic of lush greens, browns and blues. The grass is as green and as smooth as a pool table. I am out for a 7 am ride on Euripides and get to the point on the mile-long bridleway called Rotten Row that is closest to the Serpentine, the lake in Hyde Park, when Euripides decides to turn right, walk a hundred feet across the grass, put his forelegs in the Serpentine and have a long drink. Embarrassing but fine. Then he refuses to budge. I put him in reverse. Nothing. I spur him forward. He just stands there, forelegs in two feet of water, hind legs on the paving, staring across the lake. It is as if he wants to breathe in the sheer beauty of a wonderful morning.

Cavalrymen from nearby Hyde Park Barracks, a thirty-three-storey eyesore that opened at the same time I started working for Brian two years previously, canter by and wave. Euripides doesn't notice or seem to have a care in the world. Even though I'll have to dismount into the water, I am just about to get off and lead my horse back to the bridleway when a woman wearing a black top hat, in a grey jacket and ankle-length dress, riding side saddle, approaches my right side. *Side saddle!*

'Good morning. I see you have been here for some time and wondered whether there was a problem,' she comments.

This is embarrassing. I'm sitting on a horse that refuses to move, and a women riding by has seen and understood my predicament.

'Dr Fogle! What a pleasant surprise to meet you here. I didn't know you had a horse.'

I have no idea who she is.

'Good morning. Yes, Euripides' owner lets me ride him. I don't very often, but when the weather is as wonderful as this I try to get out here at least once every two weeks.'

'It's Biddy Abbott,' she replies, seeing the vacant look in my face. 'Rabbit's mother, that foolish Jack you so brilliantly diag-nosed with lead poisoning. Is Euripides playing "statue"?'

'Well, I think he's contemplating the beauty of the morning as much as I have been, and yes, he's turned into a statue,' I reply.

Brian had mentioned she lived in Buckingham Palace, and I wondered whether that had anything to do with the way she was dressed or why she was riding side saddle. I don't ask, but it is obvious she is a skilled horsewoman.

'If you hand me the reins, I'll lead him out,' Mrs Abbott explains, and elegantly she backs her horse from my right side and walks to my left and now, with her horse almost touching mine and her back to me, she reaches over, takes Euripides' reins and walks her horse forward. Euripides doesn't follow. He stands, continuing to contemplate the meaning of life.

'Dr Fogle, do you mind if I speak directly to Euripides?' Mrs Abbott asks, and I say, 'Please do.'

With the reins still in her right hand, Mrs Abbott looks over her right shoulder and in a voice that is probably heard on the thirty-third floor of the Barracks says, 'Euripides, move your fucking arse now!' He does.

I grin at her ease with vulgarity, thank her, and after returning Euripides to his stables, walk to Pont Street, where I learn
that an hour earlier another dog, this time a young Basset
hound, had run into Victoria Station and electrocuted himself
on a live rail. Trains were delayed while the dog's body was
recovered from the tracks and brought to us for disposal. I
recognise Snoopy, an endearing cartoon of a dog, and ring his
owners with the dreadful news. He had been on his way to
Burton Court, opposite the Royal Hospital Chelsea, for his
morning exercise, when he bolted, pulling his lead from his
owner's hands and run off. No one could catch him. Somehow
he successfully crossed Chelsea Bridge Road, Pimlico Road and
Buckingham Palace Road before he ran to his death in the train
station.

I was of equally negligible value to the people I see that
morning, most of whom want my advice on their dogs'
behaviour. One dog screams so much when her owners go out
that the neighbours have reported them to the police. 'I
thought dogs could take care of themselves,' the West Highland
terrier's owner tells me. 'No one told me she would turn into
an emotional cripple.' I give the tepid advice I have gleaned
from Barbara Woodhouse's record and books – leave the radio
on, leave toys to play with, have her neutered. It would be
years before I could give more practical and successful
instructions.

I was on duty for the central London vets that evening,
so Julia came over and made dinner for us at Pont Street.
We talked about our living arrangements and decided that
she would tell Emily that we loved each other and that
soon I would be moving in with them. 'She'll question you
until she's blue in the face,' Julia explained, but I'd known
Emily for over a year and figured I could handle a four-year-
old's interrogation.

Julia decided to stay the night, and after the typical flurry of 11 pm calls we went to bed. At 2 am the phone rang. Julia passed it over to me. It was Margaret, Duchess of Argyll, and her Poodle Antoine was having bad dreams. She wanted and eventually demanded a home visit.

'Why do you think Antoine is having bad dreams?' I ask over the phone, and am told that he was restless and pacing around the room.

'Did he eat and drink normally?' I ask, and am told he did.

'Have you taken him out to see if he needs to pee or poo?' I ask, and am told very explicitly that he had 'spent both a penny and tuppence' before they all went to bed.

'Have you given him anything?' The Duchess told me she had given her little dog a Valium tablet, then a Mogadon tablet. Both of these drugs have a calming effect on the brain, and in people they decrease anxiety, relax muscles and increase sleepiness. She could have had them prescribed to her to treat insomnia.

'I think Antoine is fighting the effects of the pills you've given him and that's why he's pacing,' I explain, and am told that this is ridiculous, that she is alone with no one to help her and that I should come over to her house on Upper Grosvenor Street at once.

I suggest that she takes Antoine out for a walk. Jokingly, I suggest that she brews up some dark coffee for him and when I say that all hell breaks loose.

'Mr Fogle, if you do not come here at once, I will see that you lose your job and never work in London again!'

I lose it and find myself saying, 'Ah, shit. Go fuck yourself.' And I hang up.

Julia is goggle-eyed. She has never heard me swear. I don't swear. I don't like swearing. But, if you'll pardon me saying so,

I was pissed off and I explain why to Julia, who giggles when she hears the whole story.

'What are you going to tell Brian?' she says, and it's then I feel sick.

What am I going to tell my ramrod-erect, ethical, conventional and frankly scary boss?

Julia tries to distract me, but I can't help but play over in my mind how I would tell Brian what I had said to Margaret, Duchess of Argyll. What if there is something dreadfully wrong with Antoine and she has to take him to another vet? What if he dies? What if she tells Brian she's going to tell all her friends never to take their pets to Pont Street again?

On Wednesdays, Brian was at his home in Surrey, operating. I couldn't face telling him over the telephone what I had done, and with Pat's agreement – I told Pat exactly what happened, and she was shocked – I decided to tell him when he arrived for work on Thursday.

Frustratingly, Brian was delayed by traffic on Thursday, and by the time he had unloaded that week's batch of dogs ready to be returned to their homes both of us already had clients waiting in reception. I go into his office and say, 'I'll explain more later but briefly, I was impolite to one of your clients, Margaret, Duchess of Argyll, and I'm sure she'll be speaking to you about my behaviour.'

'We'll speak about this later, but briefly tell me what happened,' Brian asks.

'She demanded a home visit to see her dog, who was having bad dreams after she had given him Valium and Mogadon. I gave her advice on how to walk her dog around. She became very abusive, and I told her to go fuck herself.'

Brian turned from the medical records he was sorting through and came around his desk to me – grinning the broadest grin. He grasped my shoulders.

'Good man! I've wanted to do that for years,' he says. 'Now, let's not leave people waiting.' And he returned to his desk and buzzed reception that he was ready. As I left the room, he called me back.

'Bruce,' he says, 'I once did the same with Zsa Zsa Gabor.'

25

My relationship with Julia was heading towards permanence, so in early August, when she had a break in her schedule – rehearsals for her next play, with Deborah Kerr, would start at the beginning of September – I took her back to Canada for the tail end of my two weeks' annual holiday, this time leaving Emily and Honey in Rita's care. We flew to Toronto, picked up a rental car and drove to the family cottage on Lake Chemong in the Kawartha Lakes, to spend the holiday break with my parents.

Things got off to a bad start. Julia couldn't cope with the heat and humidity. 'It's like someone's opened an oven door!' she exclaimed as we exited the plane and walked down the gangway onto the searing tarmac, then into the airless terminal building. She wilted. I was used to the sultry, humid Gulf of Mexico weather that each summer funnels up the Mississippi River valley and envelops southwestern Ontario in a sweaty, energy-sapping fug. Air conditioning in cars or homes was still a rare luxury, so we drove the hundred miles to the cottage with all the windows down in the car. It was 103 degrees Fahrenheit, over 39 degrees Celsius, but with high humidity it felt far hotter. By the time we got to the cottage Julia had a migraine and, after a perfunctory hello, went to her room to lie down, staying there until the following morning. From my mother's viewpoint, this was treason.

While Julia rested and her head pounded, I went for a swim, and as I dried myself off on the front lawn, my mother comes out of the cottage.

'She's certainly not very sociable,' she says sternly.

'The heat's got to her and she's got a terrible migraine,' I reply. 'She did a six-month run in a play, then went straight into a film and finished last week. She's just had a transatlantic flight and her body is exhausted.'

I could see by the set of my mother's jaw that this was not an acceptable excuse.

'If she is so exhausted, then perhaps it would have been better for her to stay at home.'

For the last forty years, until my mother died at one hundred years of age, she embraced Julia in a bone-shattering hug each time they met, looked her straight in the eye and uttered the same mantra. 'You see how wrong I was?' Julia would smile, shrug her shoulders and endure the lung-compressing embrace. In the summer of 1972, it was a different story. As far as I could tell, my mother simply didn't like Julia and didn't want her to be there. I didn't know why.

Ice formed in the oppressive heat. I was too insipid to do much, other than commiserate with Julia, who saw how she was being treated and bristled. Now there were two unaccommodating, blonde billy goats in a head-to-head encounter, neither interested in understanding the other.

We were there for two weekends and the week in between, and rather than confront the problem I did what I always did and opted out. After a short stay at the cottage, we left for Quebec City on what I told my parents was a pre-planned whale-watching trip. That re-energised both of us, and we returned to the cottage to find my brother Rob and sister-in-law Eileen, and, unexpectedly, my Uncle Reub and his wife Cynthia.

My mother had stewed during the days we were away. On our return, she almost immediately takes me to her car, sits me in it and tells me bluntly I should have nothing to do with Julia.

'If you're thinking about marrying that woman, think hard,' she says.

'Mum, we're more than good friends,' I reply.

'Don't interrupt when I'm talking. I know you are. That's why I'm telling you to think twice about getting yourself into a hopeless situation!'

'Mum, listen,' I reply and she retorts, 'Don't you "Mum, listen" me. Don't talk back to your mother!'

I give up, get out of the car and march off. Respect your parents. I was taught that from the time I could think. Part of me wants to cry. Part of me wants to murder her.

I walk for half an hour, then suddenly worry that my mother might be confronting Julia, and race back to the cottage, where Julia, Eileen, Uncle Reub and his wife Cynthia are on lounge chairs in the front garden by the lake, chattering and drinking. Julia sees the tenseness in my face, comes over and asks if I am all right. I explain I'd had a disagreement with my mother and joined the gathering.

'Bruce has had a contretemps with his mother,' Julia announces, a bit sensationally.

'Over what?' Eileen asks, but rather than tell them I ask Uncle Reub if we could, as we had done many times before, go for a walk. As we stroll down the gravelled road I tell him that my mother has, in effect, told me to choose between Julia and her.

We walk in silence, until Uncle Reub stops by a neighbour's cottage. No one is there, and he invites me to sit with him on the two swings hanging from a tree by the road.

'Let me tell you something about my kid sister,' Uncle Reub begins. 'Everything she does she does out of love, although that may not be evident to you at this moment.'

We both swing gently on our swings.

'You know that our parents died when your mother was young and this is something she never got over. For her entire life she has felt abandoned and, as good as your father is to her, she still feels abandoned.'

'You're telling me this is why she dislikes Julia?' I ask.

'Yes it is, but let me first tell you about your parents,' Reub replies.

'Your father. He was raised to avoid any show of emotion. It's not manly to show emotion. But you know he would die for you. Your mother. She loved you even before she met you. And after she met you and you grew to be the person you are, she loved you even more. Bruce, you know we both lack a belief in religion, so when I say she wants you to be her god, you know what I mean. She confides in you. Since you were ten years old she's relied on you for emotional support. And now, because she sees you are serious about Julia, she fears being abandoned by you.'

'Uncle Reub, that's an attractive way to put it, but it's too intellectual. She just doesn't like Julia,' I say.

'If it were that simple, she wouldn't get so emotional,' Reub answers.

He continues. 'I didn't understand my own behaviour with women. I'm not exaggerating when I say that that's why I left ear, nose and throat, and qualified as a psychiatrist. And Bruce, I've learned that there is a universal dimension to human behaviour, and that is that we unwittingly create the fate we fear. We behave in thoughtless ways and end up exactly where we don't want to be. Your mother doesn't want to lose you and her behaviour is increasing that possibility. She's not going to let go of you. So you're going to have to let go of her. You may not know it, but your moving to London two years ago was the start. Did you do so intentionally, to put a body of water between the two of you?'

'I never thought that moving to England was because I wanted to break free from Mum's clutches.'

'Bruce, I like to think of life in physical terms. Your accomplishments in life, and I know you will have many of them, they will seem to others to be yours. But that simplifies life. Who you are and what you do in your life rests on top of your parents' stories and their parents' stories and their parents' stories. During your lifetime you are the stone on top of the pyramid. And you are fortunate, my boy, to reside on such a firm foundation.'

'Uncle Reub,' I reply, 'you're as corny as Mum is. Okay. I get what you're saying. I don't know if that makes her behaviour any easier.'

Years later, when I asked my mother why she was so vitriolic – was it that Julia was an actress, or had a child, or wasn't Jewish – she told me she was venomous because she thought Julia 'wasn't good enough for me'. When I asked her what she meant by that she said, 'I don't really know. As a child you meant so much to me, you were the one person I could always talk to. You still are. I don't think anyone would have been good enough.'

26

It was my first day back at work and Christopher was distraught. The country had experienced another national dock strike, yet another State of Emergency, a British Rail work to rule and now there was a newspaper strike, but Christopher was breathless because he had just run from his shop to the surgery with the limp body of a Scottie in his arms.

'I found it like this in the drying cabinet.'

There was no need for me to listen with my stethoscope. The dog's eyes were widely dilated and its gums were white.

'What happened?' I ask.

'It was simply in for a shampoo. The girls washed him and put him in the drying cabinet. I don't know why, but I decided to check on the dogs. The others were fine and this one was curled up as if he was sleeping. When he didn't look up at me, I picked him up and he was as limp as a rag. That's when I ran over here.'

'If he was just lying there, it sounds like he lay down and died,' I comment. I poked the Scottie's belly and felt a fluid roll, got a syringe and needle, inserted it and drew out fresh blood.

'Something haemorrhaged in here. Probably the liver or the spleen. Do you want me to do a post-mortem?'

'I dread it but yes, once I find his owner and get permission. Oh god, I have to take a dog to Orly later today. The owner asked the mother to deliver the dog but will have to make do with the son.'

'Can you postpone until this evening?' I ask.

'I'm on the last Air France flight,' Christopher replies. 'And only Air France lets dogs travel in the passenger section, as long as you buy a full-price ticket for it. I wonder if my stepfather will take it? Oh god. I hate this business.'

Christopher went back to his shop, I went back to my list of consultations and an hour later he was on the telephone to me.

'Yes, please do a post-mortem. We have the owner's permission. All he said was, "Oh dear. What a pity. Do you have any Scottie pups?" But *I* need to know what happened. And my stepfather is taking the Shih Tzu to Orly, so let me know what happened once you know.'

'Nag's Head at 7 pm, then,' I reply.

We meet at seven. The air is damp, so we sit down inside.

'Ruptured liver,' I tell him. 'Sudden, catastrophic blood loss. There would have been some discomfort from all that blood in the abdomen, but even if I'd been there when it happened there's nothing I could have done to save him.'

'What do you think happened?' Christopher asks.

'My hunch is he tried to jump out of the sink, bashed his belly in exactly the wrong place and tore his liver.'

We drank from our glasses.

'God, I hate this business,' Christopher continues. 'Mother's leaving. My mother and stepfather love living in Cornwall so the business is mine, and I hate it. Do you know how you stumble into doing things, not because you plan it but because stuff just happens? The dogs are great. Most of the buyers are great too. But running a shop? I never wanted to be a shopkeeper. Arguing with landlords. Challenging the rates. Neighbours complaining about noise. Dogs dying when they're shampooed. I could shut down the shop and be just as successful as a finder. I don't need all this aggravation. Bruce, are you listening?'

Christopher saw my mind was elsewhere. I was listening but I was thinking about my being in London, doing what I was doing, not because I'd made intentional plans but just because 'stuff happens'. The travel scholarship had been a random event. I'd mentioned zoo animal medicine to the associate dean, not because I was interested in it but because it was the first thing that came into my mind. I stayed in London passively, because Brian offered me a job, not because I went out looking for one. I was now deeply involved with Julia because she invited me out. Christopher rabbited on about his ideas for a bespoke 'concierge' dog-finding and dog-boarding service, and I was finally thinking about what I was going to do with my life.

27

'Bruce, this is Bryan O'Breen. I met Bryan while you were visiting your parents, and he will be joining the practice while I am in Guelph.'

'G'day. Call me Bluey,' the new arrival grinned, and he gave me a two-handed handshake.

Bluey had a naturally happy face, freckled, curtained with lustrous ginger hair. His green eyes danced with waywardness. You know how you make instant judgements? Mine was that I thought this would be a great guy to go on a pub crawl with, but would I put the welfare of my dog in his hands?

'Professor Blood at Melbourne tells me Bryan, who was one of his students, is a superb surgeon. He will undertake the orthopaedic surgery in my absence, of course under your supervision, Bruce. You are responsible for decision-making while I'm away.'

I knew of the aptly named Douglas Blood. While he was at my college, with another of my professors, Jim Henderson, he wrote the most vital veterinary textbook of its time, the simply titled *Veterinary Medicine*.

Brian continued, 'As you are no longer using the flat upstairs, I've told Bryan he can use it while he is here. Is that acceptable to you, Bruce?'

Bruce, Bryan, Brian. For a moment it crossed my mind we sounded like an Australian pop group, but then I looked at my boss Brian and returned to reality.

'Yes. Absolutely.'

'Bryan, I'd like to speak with Bruce privately for a moment. Pat will show you around your accommodation.'

Bluey left the room and Brian looked relaxed. Sitting on the edge of his desk, he told me he wanted me to stay on after he returned from his sabbatical, as his permanent assistant.

'I know you have planned to return to Canada, but you are an excellent veterinary surgeon, clients tell me you are good to their pets and I think we make a first-rate team. Your salary will be a guaranteed minimum plus a share of the profits. It will be equivalent to your becoming a partner, without any of the nuisances of ownership.'

I felt as pleased as I ever had, and told Brian I was grateful for the offer and we'd discuss it through letters while he was in Guelph. But I had immediate worries. One was that this would be yet again my making a decision because an opportunity dropped into my lap, rather than my making a decision, then looking for opportunities. The other was that I came from a culture where you were your own boss. My father and all of my uncles, professionals and shopkeepers, were self-employed. They did the employing. My knee-jerk assumption was that after being employed by someone I'd put up my own plate, be my own boss. Brian was offering me virtually guaranteed employment and a share of the profits, but not decision-making. If I were to stay, I knew that's what we'd have to discuss in our letters.

For the rest of the week all three of us worked at the surgery, with Bluey alternately shadowing Brian or me. I'm sure that when Bluey shadowed Brian he asked medical and surgical questions, but when he shadowed me he asked about the nurses, about clients and about London.

'Say mate, who are all those good-looking chicks next door?'
Bluey asks one day.

I'd noticed them too when I first started working at Pont
Street.

'Up-market call girls,' I explain.

'You're kidding me, mate. They're bloody gorgeous!'

'That's why they're up-market,' I boastfully explain, pleased
that I could be so blasé, so metropolitan, about such things.

Brian departed for Canada and I was, at least technically, in
charge. I felt that I should be in the surgery as much as possible,
so I told Bluey he would be doing the home visits.

'No sweat, mate.'

I also wanted to see what his surgical skills were like and asked
him to do all the surgery in his first full week at Pont Street.

'No sweat, mate.'

Brian was absolutely right. Bluey was a confident surgeon
with natural skills. We saw a dog that week with a peach stone
lodged for so long where the small intestine meets the large
intestine that that section of intestine had to be removed and
the healthy bits reconnected, not the easy way, which is end to
end, but the more complicated way, side to side. I watched and
envied his dexterous hands.

On the first Friday of our working alone together, just before
afternoon appointments began, Bluey piled into my room.

'Fuck me! Look at this mate,' he roars as he pulls up his shirt
and shows me massive bruising from his waist to his left
shoulder.

'That home visit? To those bloody Dobies? All I did was turn
my back on them and that bitch went for me.'

I didn't get bitten by a dog until I'd been with Brian for
almost a year, and then it was only a hand puncture. This was
a really nasty attack bite.

'Sharon? In Berwick Street Market?' I ask.

'Yeah, mate. That's the one. Know her?'

I explain I did and that I was surprised that either of her dogs would bite.

'Ah, mate, she's on the game, so I didn't think she'd mind me copping a feel, but her fucking dog did!'

'Bluey, did you seriously grab her tits?'

'It was barter, mate.'

'Bluey, we're in Rome so we do as the Romans do. I don't know what it's like in Oz, but here you ask first. Okay?'

That wasn't the last of Bluey's interactions with women while he worked at Pont Street.

'Bruce, Bluey, a meeting at 8.30 tomorrow morning, please.'

When Pat was stern, frankly she was scary. Behind her back, Brenda and Annabelle called her Matron.

'Gentlemen, while Mr Singleton is away, when you are on these premises you keep your firearms in your holsters. Am I clear?'

'What?' I ask.

'Yeah, mate. I get it,' Bluey replies.

Amazingly, I don't, and after the brief meeting I follow Pat downstairs and ask, 'What's up?'

'His pecker,' she replies. 'He's knocking off just about a client a night. He might want England to be peopled only by red-headed children, but I'm not having Mr Singleton coming back to any dramas.'

'But you knew about Rose and me, and Julia and me,' I say.

'Bruce, you're a harmless amateur. Bluey is a womaniser. He's interested in notches on his pistol, not relationships.'

After work, when I meet Julia returning from her rehearsals for her next play, I tell her Bluey behaved as if it were natural to grope women.

'So does just about every actor I've ever met. If I *don't* get groped at rehearsals, I look in the mirror to see if there's something wrong.'

Julia and I had our evenings to ourselves, and once more it was the *Evening Standard*'s Pub of the Year selection. We both agreed that the Victoria in Bermondsey, a Truman's pub standing on its lonesome between a housing estate and an industrial estate, was our favourite. I'm sure that the Queen Vic in the TV soap *EastEnders* that started ten years later was named after this perfectly tiled, dark-wood-panelled Victorian masterpiece.

With a live-in nanny, we had most evenings free. We visited Julia's friends Frank and Jackie frequently. Frank told Julia he had an idea for another play he wanted to write for her. It would be called *Blind Date*.

We had dinner with Diana and Morogh Balfour and were enchanted with their stories of Venice, where, they told us, they went for their honeymoon, and every year since for all of August. They took Mark, their butler, with them, and while they stayed with friends, Mark was given accommodation in a nearby pension. When we left, Morogh, escorted us to the front door, then handed Julia two candelabras I had noticed standing on a side table.

'These are for you,' Morogh beams.

'They are gorgeous, but Morogh, I can't take them. They're yours,' Julia replies.

'You told Diana how beautiful you thought they are. You must have them,' he insists.

Julia looks at me and I give a slight affirmative nod to her.

'Morogh, if you ever invite us back, I'm looking at *nothing* other than you and Diana,' Julia says, and standing on her tiptoes she gives this elegant man a tight hug.

Driving back to Julia's home I jokingly asked her if Morogh was giving things away because he needed hugs.

'It's upsetting,' she replies. 'It's as if he's getting his house in order.'

28

In 1972, if you walked along Oxford Street anywhere near Selfridges, you would meet a long-faced, flat-capped, bespectacled man carrying a sign, '*The end of the world is nigh,*' a group of saffron-robed, shaven-headed English kids rhythmically drumming and chanting '*Hare Krishna*', and Mr Tatterby with his capuchin monkey perched on his shoulder, offering to take a photo of you with his well-mannered companion. Mr Tatterby – 'Call me Tatterby,' he told me when we met – reminded me of a grinning gecko. Although he was outdoors all day, his complexion was pasty, and when he grinned his thin lips retracted in a reptilian manner. I don't mean to be disparaging about him. I didn't like him using his monkey as a source of income, a modern variation on the organ grinder's capuchin monkey working the crowd, begging with cup in hand, but once I got to know Tatterby, he was a patently good man, a bit lost, and always on the lookout for a reliable source of income.

Dolores del Aruba, to give you her full name, his white-faced capuchin monkey, was at least fifteen years old when I met her, with yellow hair on her neck, throat and upper arms, a creamy-coloured face and a crown of black hair on her head, like a friar's cap. The rest of her hair was black. She weighed around three kilos, a hefty weight when she sat on my shoulder, with her enormously long tail wrapped comfortably around my neck. She loved strawberries in particular, was overweight and diabetic. Tatterby had brought her to the surgery six months previously because she was regurgitating her food. He mentioned in passing that she was drinking much more than usual. On that first visit, Dolores had the good sense to pee on me, giving me the opportunity to check if there was any sugar in her urine, and there was. Without doing blood tests, as I would today, I concluded she had Type II diabetes, common in captive primates. Primates living a natural life in the environment they evolved in probably never suffer from diabetes, but I had learned during my brief time working at Regent's Park Zoo that the condition was common – very common – in captive primates, regardless of whether they were in circuses, zoos, research establishments or living in people's homes as Dolores did. If a monkey was bottle-fed as an infant, lived with people and didn't get much exercise, it risked developing diabetes. And if it ate what it liked, sugary or starchy foods like bananas and strawberries or fatty foods like chips from the Sea Shell fish and chip shop on Lisson Grove, as Dolores did, diabetes was all but inevitable.

In Type II diabetes, the body continues to produce insulin; it has simply become resistant to it, so in Dolores's circumstances she didn't need twice-daily insulin injections. She needed a better diet, and Tatterby was good at this. He immediately cut out the chips, then gradually reduced the sugary fruit in her diet, replacing it with vegetable greens and occasional bits of cooked chicken breast. At the zoo the primates were given pumpkins and marrows, so I also added tinned pumpkin. It was available in Selfridges Food Halls, handy for Tatterby's 'office', the pavement outside. To be on the safe side, I told him to give Dolores a daily drop of Abidec, a concentrated vitamin supplement for infants. In fact, a dozen times a day I told people to give their pets Abidec drops. It was a habit I got into until Meredith asked me if I had ever seen a vitamin deficiency in an animal I had treated, and I couldn't think of one. Relatively new drugs called sulfonylureas, close relatives of the sulfa drugs I routinely used as antibiotics (but with no antibiotic effect themselves), were just starting to be marketed as oral agents to reduce blood sugar in people suffering from Type II diabetes, but Tatterby told me that Dolores would not take kindly to being forced to swallow pills.

Now Dolores was back in the surgery, and I knew why. She had started to develop abscesses around her fingernails. Sometimes she bit the boils to release the pus but this led to rough healing. Tatterby and I agreed that when an abscess looked ripe, he'd bring Dolores in and I'd lance it and clean it. She didn't like that.

I knew that monkeys were capable of using tools; I had seen a film of a capuchin monkey pick up a stick and chase a capybara away from its food, but Dolores's use of tools was more inventive. As usual, she sat on Tatterby's shoulder as he climbed the stairs and entered my consulting room. And as I walked from behind my desk to go to the shelves above the sink to get a sterile scalpel blade to incise her abscess, she coughed, not to clear her throat but as a threat, then stood up, dropped a hand between her legs, dropped a turd into her hand and with great accuracy threw it at me.

This was an inventive use of tools. First of all, I noted that Dolores was a right-hander and thought she'd be far more valuable as a pitcher for the New York Yankees than panhandling for Tatterby. Secondly, my quandary was what to do. I was obviously scaring her shitless, but at least she found a creative use for the physiological response to her distress.

Tatterby had watched me lance Dolores's previous abscesses and cleanse her fingers with non-stinging povidone-iodine solution and he made a suggestion.

'I think Mrs Tatterby and I can do that at home,' he explained.

Tatterby had never mentioned Mrs Tatterby to me before. I thought of him as married to a small hairy primate, not to a large hairless one.

I often saw Mr Tatterby and Dolores outside Selfridges when visiting Miss Williams's feral cats in Balderton Flats, but then a year later, when I moved to nearby Seymour Street and Selfridges became our local general store, I saw them at least weekly. Dolores happily climbed onto tourists' shoulders and examined their hair while Mr Tatterby took photos, money and addresses to send the pictures to. Then they were gone and I assumed Dolores had died. Capuchins can live forty-five years or more, but not diabetic ones. Diabetics die before their time. Years later, Julia and I chanced upon Tatterby in Arundel, West Sussex, where he and Mrs Tatterby were now working as antique dealers, and they were more anxious to tell me that Dolores was still alive than they were to sell us their antiques.

'When she slimmed down, Mrs Tatterby told me we will move to the country where Dolores can be more active,' he explained. 'Until a short time back, she always accompanied us when we went buying. Guaranteed to get us a good price. Mind you, she had a good eye for a bargain, better than either of us,' and he smiled his reptilian grin.

29

I've never had an original thought. At least not a truly original one. Not the type I had seen in researchers at university. Carlton Gyles was Student President in my first year at veterinary college, a leading research scientist by the time I was in my final year. After buying his way out of his obligation to return to his native Jamaica, he investigated bloody diarrhoea in pigs. This was expensive, and time consuming. He could only test one of the hundreds of strains of *E. coli* bacteria on one pig. But he had an original thought, acted on it, and developed a technique where he could study forty or more strains on one animal. I envied that ability, and although for a long time I thought that working with companion animals was only a temporary job, that one day I would return to university, privately I questioned my abilities to be a creative scientist.

What I learned working for Brian was to take other people's original thoughts, to listen to what they were saying, and do something about it. I was now thinking about why I was a vet. Some answers were easy. As my competence increased, so too did the satisfaction I got from doing what I do. I enjoyed being helpful to others. I don't understand why being good to others can be so satisfying, but it is. I had a new identity too and I liked that, someone who cares for animals.

But I wonder. Is it as simple as that, my enjoyment in being a vet? Perhaps it's not just the plain pleasure of making things better. Perhaps I was thinking about taking up Brian's offer, of staying in London out of the straightforward vanity that I didn't want to be just another vet, I wanted to be the best, and that would be easier in London than in North America. Is that asking too much? Maybe I thought that I can't be best in North America because there are too many vets there. But I can be best in Britain because my university training and now my first years in clinical practice had given me such a head start. Is that dishonourable? Possibly. Possibly not. I don't think it should be. Wouldn't the world be a great place if all of us tried to be masters of what we do, without feeling any petty rivalries towards our colleagues?

What I was learning through day-to-day experience was that not only did I enjoy medicine more than surgery but that I just loved mastering an understanding of why my patients behaved the way they do. Although I didn't yet know it, I was mastering new languages, understanding my patients and their owners, my patients by their body language, their owners by not just what they said but by how they said it and sometimes what they didn't say. Do you know how exciting this can be? I found myself learning the intricacies of mute communications as if they were literature. And I found, and still find, reading nature gratifying in the same way that art or music is. Watch a cat. Interpret what it's doing. Work out what it's thinking. You may say this is pure hogwash, that there's no comparison between let's say understanding a Mahler symphony and understanding why a German Shepherd wants to sit on my lap, and you're right. One is outstandingly beautiful while the other is, what can I say, cartoonish? But would you deny that as cartoonish as it is, understanding the German Shepherd's behaviour is sweetly charming, may I say even romantic?

To understand my patients I had to learn a new language, one I didn't have a single lecture in at college. When I first started working at Brian's my only objective was to 'do no harm', and for that I learned a simple vocabulary. In my frivolous comparison to understanding a symphony, that's the equivalent to listening to and liking the tuneful bits. But then you learn that nature has its own grammatical laws, set down both by evolution and where the dog or cat finds itself living. It's the same with the symphony. Where did Mahler's symphony evolve from and how did the environment in which he was writing influence his music? Is there hidden meaning you only understand through repeated listening, through discussing the music with others? Do you mind if I carry on with this pretentious comparison? To understand why a dog or cat behaves as it does, to get to that beautiful point where you understand it, where you are now mutely communicating, I found I had to travel first through what is meaningful, how ear position can vary, how whiskers can sweep out and back. Only then could I start to interpret what animals say with their bodies.

Another thing. Why was I in London? That was simple serendipity. But if Julia and I were going to spend the rest of our lives together, should we do so where her work was or in Canada, where my family was? I had questions to answer and was good at avoiding them.

30

The raw emotions, the depth of feeling people experience when pets die, can bring a disarming honesty to what they say. This was greater than I had anticipated and I certainly wasn't prepared for the intensity of emotion I saw, both when pets are ill and when the end of life arrives. When people are driven by a feeling of helplessness, of overwhelming love for their pet, some act as if they're in suspended animation, in a ghostly world of powerlessness and vulnerability.

The Admiral tried to suppress that vulnerability, but his honesty was telling. His young German Shepherd had just died in a road traffic accident. I had treated Jellicoe for fight wounds just before going to Canada with Julia and was amused by the owner's description of that dog fight. 'It was a fire and forget incident,' he told me, a perfect explanation of the type of short, snappy altercation dogs sometimes have with each other. In most instances nothing happens, but in that one Jellicoe had a tooth puncture to the skin on his neck that needed attention.

Now he was lifeless but still quite warm, having died only minutes before. The Admiral found it hard to hold back his tears but he did. With his hand buried in the hair on his dog's chest, looking at his dog, not me, he said, 'Of all my family, he was the one who never disillusioned me.'

As well as understanding why dogs and cats behave as they do, I was beginning to understand how the honesty and simplicity of animals make them so important to us. I was exposed several times a week to the searing intensity of loss, to hearing, 'I'll never get another,' almost every time a pet died, simply because the pain was so deep the pet's owner couldn't bear having to go through it again. Yet most of these people were back within the year with another pup.

Blessing was one of them, a Poodle with a purpose. Christopher had already selected Blessing for the LeBlanc's, an American family from Louisiana living in London, after their previous Poodle had died in late maturity. But before the pup arrived, Mr LeBlanc had a stroke and was bed-ridden. The new pup became his bed companion and, as far as Mrs LeBlanc was concerned, was the reason her husband improved as much as he did. That's how Blessing got her name.

'Hello, mate,' Bluey shouted as he tumbled down the stairs from his flat above the examination rooms. 'How many cats to neutralise today? You know there were four that needed bloody splaying yesterday. If they can't get their words right, why can't the Brits just say "de-sex" the way we do?'

I couldn't answer that, but Julia's play, *The Day After the Fair*, had just opened and I asked Bluey if he'd like to see it and have dinner with us afterwards. I organised a ticket for him and arranged to meet him at the stage door.

Julia's reviews were, as always, terrific. When she read in *Plays & Players*, 'the all-time sex symbol of the age, Miss Foster is becoming typecast as sex incarnate, and she is bloody good,' she put down the magazine, went nose to nose with me, and said, 'Do you ever say that to me?'

Later that evening, I met Bluey at the Lyric Theatre's stage door and waiting beside him was the American actor James Stewart. I tried to be nonplussed but I couldn't. I just stared. Up. He's a tall man.

'Do you know who that was?' I asked Bluey when we got to Julia's dressing room.

'No. Who?' he replied.

'*Mr Smith Goes to Washington. The Philadelphia Story. It's a Wonderful Life, Harvey, Anatomy of a Murder, Rear Window, Vertigo.*'

'Is he an actor then, mate?'

Julia looked at me and shrugged. She'd met Bluey before and I'd spoken highly of his professional skills so she was comfortable saying out loud, 'Well, at least he's a good surgeon.'

We went to Carroll's for the usual salt beef sandwiches, French fries and Cokes, and talked theatre.

'You were booshit, Jules!' Bluey exclaims, giving her a warm and genuine hug before we sit down, and I learn in an instant why every client was happy to climb into his bed.

'How do you do that each night?' he continues. 'You're sexy. You need a man. Any man would want to protect you. Mind you, your lady's a bit of a pearler herself. I didn't know who she was until I read the programme. Why's she here on stage in London rather than in Hollywood?'

'Because Hollywood is run by men who can only think with their willies. Debs just turned fifty, so they think it's inconceivable any man will still find her sexy. You did,' Julia answers.

'Too true, mate,' he replies.

I dropped Bluey off at the surgery and continued home with Julia, who was quiet and pensive.

As we enter her flat, she turns to me and says, 'Part of me loved the *Plays & Players* review, but a bigger part of me hated it. Isn't it sad that someone with Deborah's talents is discarded because she's not considered as sexy as she once was. I don't want to be known for being sexy. I want to be known for being a serious actress.'

31

It was late November. The first frost of winter had arrived and it was a time of year when dogs don't get 'summer dermatitis', but on Saturday evening Julia's dog Honey developed a bothersome patch of moist skin infection below her ear. When I got up on Sunday morning it was much worse, so before breakfast I borrowed Julia's Mini and drove over to Pont Street to get clippers, antiseptic and a tube of 'mastitis ointment', procaine penicillin in a squeezable tube.

As I unlocked the front door to the surgery, Brenda appeared on the stairs in her negligee, then quickly disappeared back upstairs.

Shit. Bluey's now charming the knickers off the staff.

'G'day, mate!' he shouts down the stairs. 'Need any help?'

'Hi. It's okay. I'm just picking up some stuff for my dog.'

'Stay for breakfast, mate,' Bluey counters.

'Thanks, but I'd better get back to the dog,' I reply.

Brian was expected back on Monday morning. We'd exchanged two letters during his absence. In his first he wrote out details of our planned relationship. I would make all decisions on the medical side of the practice – equipment we should buy, drugs to use, clinical tests to carry out. I liked that. Often we were still making our own ointments and unguents.* The microscope I used to examine stained slides was older than I was. Brian still preferred to treat worm infestations with purgatives that caused explosive diarrhoea. If his offer was genuine, I'd have, for example, the authority to switch entirely to the new parasite-control drugs that killed worms without causing intestinal upset.

Brian would retain responsibility for the surgical and business sides of the practice. He would ask my opinion on hiring and firing but he'd make those decisions. He would continue to be responsible for financial decisions, although again he would discuss major questions such as expansion of the business with me.

I discussed his proposal with friends. After considering all the pros and cons, I told him that I appreciated his offer but would like the right to become a part-owner of the business at a set time in the future written into our agreement. Brian replied that he understood my request and that it was a sensible one, but that it placed too much of a restriction on any future decisions he might want to make. He explained he was returning a few weeks earlier than planned. In turn, I wrote to him that I enjoyed working for him but that one day I would like to be my own boss.

Brian wasn't the only person in Canada I was getting letters from. As well as the usual letters from my immediate family, I received two from my mother's brothers Bill and Sam. Both cautioned me against marrying Julia. I didn't hear from Ed, the brother she was closest to. I was sure she would have asked him too to write on her behalf, so I knew both Ed and Reub disagreed with her attempts to control my life. Those letters,

---

* Oily ointments. At that time many large-animal products were called unguents. The words 'unguent' and 'ointment' are interchangeable.

however, firmed my resolve that if I were to marry Julia I'd want it to be a happy event, and that meant not having my mother at it. I thought about Uncle Reub's comment that unwittingly we create situations we fear most and for a moment felt sorry for my mother, then thought, *Tough shit!*

The premises were pristine for Brian's return and, although it was a dank December morning, he arrived looking relaxed and with his usual punctuality, although there were no appointments for him. Pat had ensured he'd have the day to catch up on paperwork, make telephone calls and write essential letters.

With Brian back there were three vets at the surgery and a workload for not much more than one and a half. Bluey stayed on doing most of the surgery that month before his planned return to Australia to spend Christmas with his family. I took Brian and his wife Hilda to see Julia in *The Day After the Fair*, and the four of us had dinner at Drones afterwards, where Brian surprised me with a plan I didn't see coming.

'Bruce, I discovered when I was President of the Royal College of Veterinary Surgeons that I have administrative abilities. What surprised me is how satisfying that work can be. In Guelph, I realised that I have immense respect for researchers. They are fortunate at Guelph. Dennis Howell knows how to raise money for research and Jim Archibald understands how to use it wisely. For a long time John Hodgman has wanted me to join the Animal Health Trust. That brilliant surgery they did last year on Mill Reef, the champion racehorse? I want to ensure they have funding to do much more than that. I think I can be more useful at the Trust than at Pont Street, so next year I will become their new Director. I'm selling the practice and you are the first to know.'

I didn't realise that he was giving me first option to buy his business, so I said, 'That sounds really exciting. What do you plan to do with Pont Street?' and Hilda interjected, 'Bruce,

Brian would like you to buy the surgery. He knows it will be in safe hands.'

'Wow. Thanks. That sounds amazing. How do we go about that?' Brian told me there was a veterinary surgeon who valued surgeries and that a valuation would be arranged. I could do the same if I wished.

'Thanks. No, I won't need to do that if you know someone who does,' I replied.

Julia squeezed my hand. She was excited by the prospect of my owning Pont Street.

'While we wait for the valuation, I'll get the last three years' accounts for you to look at so you can see the profitability of the business. While you have been here it has risen each year.'

That week Brian gave me bound copies of the accounts for the years ending in April 1970, 1971 and 1972. I had never before looked at accounts, but could still see his bottom-line profit was an awful lot more than I was being paid as a salaried vet. I took them immediately to my friend David, whom I considered knowledgeable in financial matters. David looked at them for no more than a couple of minutes, then turned to me and said, 'Do you know the yearly rent for Pont Street is no more than your weekly salary? That must be the best property bargain in London.' David asked me to find out why the rent was so low and Brian explained that Woody, as Lady Cadogan's godson, paid what he called a 'peppercorn' rent, essentially nothing. As long as Woody was associated with the surgery, the Cadogan Estate would retain the low rent.

David told me that a 'true' or market rent rather than a 'peppercorn' rent should be included in any valuation. It wasn't. David told me I could find out directly from the Cadogan Estate what the market rent would be. I asked Keith for his advice.

Then and now, Keith knows everything that's happening within the veterinary community in London. Just as he knew that Frank had offered me a job, he knew that Brian had accepted the Directorship of the Animal Health Trust.

'Is a lease a good investment?' he questioned. 'Why don't we get together with Richard and discuss a large clinic for all of us?' Richard Halliwell was a friend presently teaching at the vet school in Cambridge. He had worked at Pont Street in the 1960s and clients filled me in with stories of how marvellous he was. The thought of working with Keith and Richard in large premises was exciting.

Did Brian sense I actually had reservations about buying the practice? I don't know. Did he know that Keith and Richard and I might jointly work together? Possibly. And if he did, he surely wouldn't have been pleased. Keith always knew all the veterinary gossip, but Brian was as well placed as anyone in our profession to know what we were thinking, let alone doing.

Whatever the reality, I decided I'd prefer to set up my own clinic rather than buy one, although I didn't know exactly where or when or how to do that. The 'when' was decided not long after, as Bluey told me he was buying the business. Hedging his bets, Brian had also given Bluey copies of the accounts. 'Where did he find the money to buy the place?' Julia asked. I didn't have an answer, but thought that with his winning ways, Bluey might have met some money during his short time in London rather than having it waiting in an Australian bank.

Bluey was a great guy, but I sure wasn't going to work for him, so I handed in my resignation, agreeing to stay until late January, giving Bluey the chance to fly home to Australia for Christmas. Knowing I was leaving soon, I had one piece of unfinished business to attend to. Harrods. Just before Christmas I visited Mr Grimwade. We had tea and shortbread biscuits in his office.

'Mr Grimwade, I'm leaving Pont Street. That means I no longer have a vested interest in what happens in your department, so may I speak frankly with you?'

'Yes, Vet,' he replied. He looked concerned.

'The health of your pets has improved wonderfully over the last few years, but your continuing to sell wildlife is a worry. Some of your staff disapprove of Harrods selling wild animals and I have to say I agree with them.'

Mr Grimwade leaned towards me.

'They are not "wild animals", Vet. They are surplus zoo animals. We find good homes for them.'

'Is a flat off the Kings Road really a good home for a lion? It doesn't matter how big its garden in Switzerland is, is it fair for a sociable animal like an elephant to be kept on its own away from other elephants, simply for the amusement of a rich person? I've listened to the nurses and none blame the people who buy wild animals from you. They blame Harrods for offering them in the first place and I agree with them. It's not good for Harrods' reputation.'

'How can you say that?' Mr Grimwade replied. 'Have you asked Harrods' customers?'

'Mr Singleton tells me the British Veterinary Association is helping the government draft an Endangered Species Act. He says it is almost certain to pass within the next two years. Harrods can be forced to stop selling wildlife, or you can take the moral high ground and make a decision to do so now.'

Grimwade crossed his arms and leaned back on his seat.

'Vet,' he replied, 'I have worked here all my adult life. I am proud of Harrods. They have been good to me. This is not my decision. It's my manager's decision and then his manager's decision.'

'I understand that,' I answered. 'What I can do is put what we're talking about into a letter for you to give to your boss.

I'm sure he'll ask you what you think, so before I do that, what do you think?

The pet department manager didn't reply at first. Then the tension in his shoulders seemed to relax. He uncrossed his arms and put a hand on each knee.

'Vet, I respect your directness and now I will be direct with you. To be honest, it has troubled me since I arrived in the pet department. But it is not for someone like me to object to what Harrods does.'

'But if you, the most experienced and knowledgeable person in the store doesn't object, who will? I asked.

Grimwade fell silent once more, but didn't take his eyes off mine. Then he said, 'Write the letter, Vet.'

32

Christmas was on a Monday in 1972. Bluey flew to Australia the previous weekend, and Brian and I worked at the surgery until the Friday before the four-day holiday weekend. I told him about the letter I was writing to Harrods, and without my asking he not only offered to co-sign it but said it would be most effective if it went on his letterhead, and he signed it as the former President of the Royal College of Veterinary Surgeons.

'Well done, Bruce,' he says. 'This should have stopped years ago.'

We cancelled the Saturday morning opening hours that weekend. London was already empty, and Keith and Andrew Carmichael were covering for us on Saturday and Sunday respectively, so I had the weekend free. I spent part of Saturday morning shifting clients' Christmas gifts from Pont Street over to Julia's flat on nearby Old Brompton Road – Harrods and Fortnum & Mason hampers, whisky, brandy, champagne and an enormous piece of ornamental white coral from John Gielgud and Martin Hensler.

Julia, of course, had matinee and evening performances on Saturday, and after lunch, while Jim exercised Honey, I took Emily to Santa's Grotto at Harrods. It was a fairly short visit because Marvin Liebman, Julia's producer, was having a

Christmas party for the cast and company in the theatre bar
between shows, where he supplied everyone with caviar and
champagne. Partners and friends were invited, although the
only other partner who came was Deborah's husband Peter
Viertel, an athletically handsome man in his early fifties.

Marvin, small, with rounded features and a naturally happy
face, hovered over his productions. Although only twenty years
older than Julia, Marvin mothered his company. And he mothered me, too. When Julia and other members of the cast came
down with colds a month previously, he brewed chicken soup
for everyone and supplied Julia with an extra Mason jar of it
for me. Julia still uses his recipe. He was always at the theatre
and invariably had someone interesting to introduce me to. He
introduced me to Peter.

'Bruce, Peter may be a wonderful author and successful playwright – he did John Huston's final screenplay for *African
Queen* with Humphrey Bogart and Kathryn Hepburn – but his
mother Salka Viertel was the most effervescent and beautiful
woman in Hollywood, and Greta Garbo's best friend.'

'And she lives with us in Klosters in Switzerland,' Peter
adds.

When Marvin 'presented' me to anyone, there was always a
reference to someone or something I'd know.

'Bruce, this is Miss Nancy McLarty from Vero Beach, Florida.
Nancy is one of my theatrical angels. She is close to the Coca-
Cola Pembertons of Atlanta, Georgia.'

'Bruce, this is my dear friend Lee Annenberg. Lee's Uncle
Harry founded Columbia Pictures. Lee is a dear friend of
Deborah's. Her husband Walter is our Ambassador.'

Marvin seemingly knew everyone, although I didn't learn the
unexpected reason why until the day Julia and I married.

On Sunday we had Christmas lunch at Julia's parents' home
in Sussex a day early so that I could cover for central London's

vets on Christmas Day. Julia, Emily, Honey and I travelled down to Sayers Common, just north of Brighton, early on Sunday morning.

If the American painter Norman Rockwell had ever painted in England he would have painted that lunch, Julia's aproned mother Jean carrying in the turkey with her husband Dick behind her, carving knife in hand. Julia's stern grandmother Matt sitting solemnly with a pink paper party hat on her head. Julia's sister Alex giving her father instructions on how best to carve the turkey, Emily having a sulk because she got over-excited then got reprimanded, Julia beaming, with dangling Christmas tree earrings and a red silk wreath with tiny bells on her head, pine branches on the window sills, mistletoe hanging from the ceiling fixture, holly from the garden on the dining room table, Honey asleep under the table, her parents' Beagle Wickham sitting – well, begging – beside Dick. I thought it was enchanting. We left her parents' home early in the evening, to get Emily in bed at a reasonable time and for me to be at Pont Street for the 8 am handover from Andrew.

On Christmas morning Andrew telephoned, to make sure I was there before he went off duty, and to update me on Brian's patients he had seen and other animals that might need continuing attention.

'Quiet until the evening,' he explains. 'Just typical vomiting and diarrhoea dogs, but then of all things a cat that had fallen into a caustic soda tank. I had them bathe it in vinegar and water for fifteen minutes, but it had already licked itself so there are mouth burns. And it's blind. You won't be able to save its eyes. They're bringing it over now for you to treat during the day. Sweet cat. Oh, and the diabetic cat that belongs to your client Dr Samuelson, it's dying of renal failure. I gave it loads of subcut fluids, and he's telephoning too and will bring her over if he remembers. Delightful man. Wonderful stories about being a society doctor before antibiotics. Is he deaf or senile?' I explained that Dr Samuelson repeated himself and made notes of our conversations because he was developing senile dementia and he knew it.

Everyone who telephoned apologised first for bothering me on Christmas Day. Many of those with animals that did need attention arrived with mince pies or boxes of chocolates.

Frank Manolson's client with the cat that had fallen into caustic soda was not in fact the cat's owner. He owned a business in Fulham that stripped painted doors back to bare pine, a fashionable change in the early 1970s. The stray cat had been able to get out of the tank by scrambling up the doors that were in it but when the tank's owner heard a commotion in his backyard, went out and saw the cat licking itself, he knew exactly what had happened.

Andrew had given painkillers, but this morning the burns were worse. The cat's tongue was literally falling apart. Alkali burns are horrific. I euthanised the poor thing. Not a happy way to start Christmas Day.

Late morning was quiet, so I telephoned Julia and she came over with Honey, who, in her calm, affable way just lay down and went to sleep, and Emily, who amused herself by pretending she was a dog, parking herself in a kennel and barking until, as she instinctively knew, she'd get our attention.

'Thanks, Em. You do a great impression of a dog. Do you think you can do a sleeping cat just as well?' Almost five years old, she was still young enough to hear the text and miss the subtext.

Julia brought a bottle of champagne, a tin of Sevruga caviar – Martin had given everyone in his play a tin of caviar – and two very small bone spoons to eat the caviar straight from the tin. I hadn't yet told her I really preferred ginger ale and pretzels, so while we waited for a client to arrive with her Yorkie who was refusing to eat, Julia opened both the bottle and the tin and we celebrated Christmas together.

The Yorkshire terrier, Amber, was a big girl, over four kilos, and she had an easy to diagnose, dangerous but simple to correct problem, a discharging womb infection.

The story I was told might have been lifted straight from an undergraduate textbook. Amber had been in season three weeks previously, had 'not been herself' for over a week, was drinking more than normal, eating less, until today she refused to eat, and had a pus-like vaginal discharge. When I took her temperature it was elevated. Today, I can treat this type of womb infection with a hormone injection and antibiotics, and delay surgery until the dog is no longer toxic, but that hormone injection was still thirty years in the future, so the only option was to operate as soon as possible.

'Oh god, of all days,' Amber's owner, a stunning Vanessa Redgrave lookalike mutters. 'Will she be back for Christmas dinner?'

'Yes, but she'll be so dopey she'll look like she's consumed all your Christmas punch,' I answer.

After Amber's owner leaves, I tell Julia I'll telephone Pat, who is on call if I need a nurse.

'What will Pat do?' Julia asks, and I explain that she would raise a vein in Amber's leg so that I can attach a 'butterfly' canula through which I'll give saline and the anaesthetic, then she'll answer the telephone while I do the emergency ovariohysterectomy.*

'I can do that!' Julia confidently replies.

I give Amber sedative and painkilling injections, and, with Julia and Emily intently watching, lay out the surgical

---

* Removal of both the ovaries and uterus.

instruments, set up the intravenous drip and fill a syringe with one-quarter-strength anaesthetic.

'What is Bruce going to do to the dog?' Emily asks her mother.

'The dog has a bad part inside her that's making her ill, so Bruce is going to remove it and make her feel better.'

Emily turns to me.

'When I have a tummy ache, can you remove it so it goes away?'

'This is a bit different, Em,' I reply. 'When you have a tummy ache it always goes away on its own, or it does if you take a little medicine. This dog will actually die unless the bad part inside her is removed.'

'If she dies, can I touch her?' Emily asks. 'I've never touched anything dead.'

'She won't die, darling,' Julia interjects. 'Bruce is going to make her better.'

'But if she does die, can I bury her?' Emily continues.

'She doesn't belong to us, so it's not for us to decide what happens to her,' Julia responds.

Emily continues. 'If it's not up to us, then why is Bruce going to remove her bad part?'

'Because Bruce is an animal doctor, and only animal doctors know how to operate and make animals better. Would you like to be an animal doctor one day?'

'No,' Emily answers and I ask why.

'Because it's boring being here,' she replies.

'Okay. Ready,' I say to Julia, who sternly tells Emily not to ask any more questions until allowed to do so.

Of all breeds of dogs, Yorkshire terriers have the best front-leg veins. They are large in diameter, straight, just under the skin and there's no downy hair getting in the way of finding them, just thin, silky guard hair that virtually disappears when the leg is cleaned with alcohol. I show Julia how pressing her finger on the front of Amber's elbow raises the vein for me and I insert the butterfly canula, have Julia release her finger, then tape the canula to Amber's leg. Julia doesn't seem to mind the blood that drips from the canula before I put a cap on it. Emily is amazingly quiet.

With the canula secured, I attach Amber's intravenous drip then add her anaesthetic, literally drops at a time; seriously ill animals need much less anaesthetic than healthy ones, and she slips into unconsciousness.

I instruct Julia how to hold Amber's head up while I put an endotracheal tube, for oxygen and gas anaesthetic, down her windpipe.

'Doesn't that hurt?' Emily asks, and I explain it doesn't hurt and also means she can breathe easily while she's asleep.

'Let's go now, darling,' Julia coaxes, and they both go upstairs while I position Amber for surgery then scrub up.

The operation, which was uncomplicated, took no more than half an hour, and during that time Julia answered two calls, one of which she was able to relay advice on what to do for a dog with Christmas Day diarrhoea and the other from Dr Samuelson. I asked Julia to book an appointment for him at 1 pm.

After I'd finished and Amber was sufficiently recovered from her anaesthetic, I returned upstairs. Julia reached up and put her arms around my neck.

'We're going now. Emily needs entertaining and Honey needs to stretch her legs. I loved helping today. I felt really useful. Will she be okay?'

'I could see by the way you set your jaw that you were throwing yourself into the role,' I reply. 'And yes, she'll go home this afternoon.'

'It wasn't a role,' Julia says. And I immediately knew it wasn't something I should have been flippant about.

'You were wonderful. You're a natural,' I say. 'When we set up our own practice I know who my first nurse will be.'

Dr Samuelson and his cat arrived by taxi at 2 pm.

'I'm so sorry to be late, Dr Fogle,' he explains. 'Of course, I wrote down the appointment time but then forgot to look at my notepad to remind myself.'

Maurice Samuelson had been a family doctor since the 1920s, with his home and surgery ten minutes' walk away, just off Sloane Square. His cat Wilberforce, although diabetic, was very heavy when I first visited. He had become thinner during the year but I still visited. He understood that I couldn't visit today.

I enjoyed those home visits. Dr Samuelson lived in a red brick Victorian mansion block. The room inside his apartment's front door was once his reception room. Now it was lifeless, with no carpet on the mosaic tiled floor and only a single chair by the entrance door, but his next room, the living room, for four decades his examination room, recapitulated his life as a doctor. The bookshelves were filled with medical texts and both ancient and present copies of the medical journal *The Lancet*. His desk was where I assumed it had always been, in the corner of the room, always littered with notes, journals and books. On it were a table lamp and beside it an examining light. The sofa and chairs were all overstuffed leather. Wilberforce looked elegant and imperious, a breathing presence that added a perfect touch to such a well lived in and comforting space.

On one on my home visits, I'd asked Dr Samuelson what was the greatest change he had seen during his time in clinical practice. I expected him to say 'antibiotics' but his answer was, 'Today the death of a single child is a tragedy. For the first part of my career the routine death of children was expected.'

When the National Health Service formed twenty-four years earlier, in 1948, Dr Samuelson willingly sold his business to it and became a full-time NHS doctor, a contractor, paid according to the number of patients he saw. He told me he was a member of CND, the Campaign for Nuclear Disarmament, and on a CND march at the Atomic Weapons Research Establishment at Aldermaston in Berkshire, had met Dr Ian Douglas-Wilson, the Editor of *The Lancet*, who had become a good friend. I'd never thought of doctors, or vets for that matter, having political opinions. We were there to diagnose and treat. But just as Dr Mort Linder, my pot-smoking, long-haired, bejewelled, hippy veterinary boss in San Francisco and his stoned friends opened my mind, Dr Samuelson's political activity made me realise that I was allowed to have political opinions. Doesn't that sound ridiculous, that it took meeting Dr Samuelson for me to appreciate this?

Each time I saw Wilberforce, Dr Samuelson would remind me, 'My last patient, you know.'

I'm sure that the diligence with which he checked his cat's blood glucose level and injected insulin every twelve hours delayed his dementia, but still, in the two years I knew him there had been a sad decline.

In the clinic I used 'Dextrostix', blood glucose test strips, to check the amount of glucose in the blood stream. On the bottle of strips was a colour chart to compare colour change to. But in his home Dr Samuelson had an 'Ames Reflectance Meter', a bulky box with a rechargeable lead battery. I didn't know such a piece of equipment existed. He had bought it the previous year, in 1971, so that he could much more accurately assess how much daily insulin to inject Wilberforce with. He inserted the Dextrostix in it and a moving pointer indicated exactly how much sugar was in the blood. He told me that as far as he was aware it was the only one in the UK that was not in a teaching hospital.

Now Wilberforce was dying from kidney failure. Andrew had forewarned me. The fluids Andrew had given the previous day hadn't helped. Wilberforce's breath had the sweet odour of terminal renal failure and he had shrunk literally to skin and bone.

'Dr Samuelson, we both know what is happening, and if you agree I think the time has come to help Wilberforce die peacefully.'

'Yes, let me see,' he replies, and gets out and reads his notepad.

'Yes, that is correct. That is exactly what Mr Carmichael told me yesterday and of course I understand. It may seem foolish, but Wilberforce knows you and I'm sure would like you to perform his last act. What do you use?' and I explain concentrated pentobarbitone.

As I draw the purple liquid into a syringe I comment, 'When I put down pets, some people tell me they'd like to have the same option their pets have, a release from suffering.'

Dr Samuelson rested both of his hands on the examination table.

'Throughout my life as a GP my patients have had that option. We use morphine. It's a family decision, husbands, wives, children and their GP. Now it's almost impossible. I keep a large bottle of phenobarb pills for myself.'

He smiles. 'I'm so forgetful I leave notes reminding me where I have hidden it.'

'I can use a tourniquet to raise a vein or if you would like I can show you how to raise it?' I offer.

'I would very much like to help. He is my last patient.'

I slipped a tourniquet onto Wilberforce's leg, just for backup, then showed Dr Samuelson how to raise the leg vein and I injected the lethal drug. His cat died quickly and there were no stressful post-death muscle twitches or contractions.

I wrapped the cat's body in a towel. There was another pet owner with her dog waiting in the reception room, but I wanted to raise the idea of his taking care of another cat, so I quickly told him about Miss Wallace's cats. To my surprise he liked the suggestion, and I told him I would telephone him once I had found out whether Miss Wallace had a relaxed stray rather than a fearful feral cat that needed re-homing.

The rest of Christmas Day was unremarkable. Dr Samuelson telephoned in the early evening to ask me if I had spoken with Miss Wallace, and I reminded him that I would do so once we were over Christmas and Boxing Day.

'Oh yes,' he replies. 'I didn't make a note of when you would contact me.'

He continues, 'Dr Fogle. Will you be there if I drop by with something?' and I tell him I will. Julia had left a full Christmas meal and I wasn't going to deny him the opportunity to express his thanks to me with mince pies or chocolates or some other Christmas goodies.

'Good evening, Dr Fogle. I no longer need this and I'm sure it will be useful to the surgery,' and he hands me two bags, one with the Reflectance Meter, the other with the battery. I know it cost the equivalent of six months' salary.

There's no way I'm leaving a clinical treasure like this for Bluey's surgery! I thought, but had the sense not to say out loud.

'If my cat is of any use to science, please do as you wish with her remains,' he continues.

'Thank you, Dr Samuelson. I appreciate your offer.'

The rest of the night was quiet. I slept in what was now Bluey's room in what would soon be his practice. The next morning I telephoned Frank Manolson to make sure he was on duty, then barrelled out of Pont Street back to Julia's with my two Harrods shopping bags, the first medical equipment for, I thought, Keith, Richard's and my large new clinic.

33

In late January 1973, I left Pont Street but already knew that Keith, Richard and I wouldn't be working together. On New Year's Day the three of us met at a pub on the A11 midway between London and Cambridge to discuss the possible partnership. Keith told me Richard had accepted a professorship at the University of Florida's vet school in Gainesville and our job was to convince him that a large, multi-man practice in the heart of London was more exciting. We failed. (Years later, Richard returned from Florida to become dean of Edinburgh's vet school, the wondrously named Royal (Dick) School of Veterinary Studies. Knowing the importance of the royal family in Britain, when I first heard this school's idiosyncratic name and was told it was 'well endowed', I thought that it was the Royal Dick, School of Veterinary Studies. The school was, in fact, established by William Dick.)

Before I left, there was one final incident at Pont Street that made me question exactly what goes on in a dog's mind. Jonathan and his working black Labrador Bess had gone pheasant shooting on the first Sunday in January on the Arundel Estate, sixty miles south of London. Even though there had been a productive shoot on the estate on Boxing Day, this one was also very productive. He told me that the eight dogs between them retrieved over 150 birds. He gave me two of them.

Pheasant shooting is what Bess lived for. It was her greatest pleasure, retrieving shot birds and not leaving even the faintest tooth mark on them. She didn't seem the least bit exhausted at the end of the shoot when Jonathan opened the back door of his Reliant Scimitar shooting brake and on command she hopped into it. She had a drink of water and fell into a deep sleep.

Jonathan stopped off at friends near Guildford for dinner and, while Bess slept, he had, he told me, an excellent meal and perhaps too much to drink. By the time he got home his wife had gone to bed so he fed Bess, but then, rather than her getting in her basket in the kitchen as she usually did, she followed him upstairs and got on their bed.

Both fell into the deepest sleep until next morning, when Jonathan's wife abruptly woke him up demanding, 'What is that dog doing on our bed?'

With twinkling eyes, Jonathan told me he explained to his wife that Bess had followed him upstairs and hopped on the bed and he just let her.

'That is *not* Bess!' she replied.

When gun dogs work they don't wear collars. And let's be frank, if you look at a row of eager-eyed, twenty-five-kilo black Lab bitches not wearing ID, can you tell one from another? On the shoot was another lean, young black Lab named Tess. That's who jumped into Jonathan's shooting brake. Bess had done the same, jumping into another of the guns' cars and that man hadn't noticed either! The men quickly traced their mistake and thought it was very amusing. Their wives didn't find it funny at all. At his wife's insistence, Jonathan brought Bess to me to make sure she had not been 'damaged' by the mistake.

For over fifty years now, my home and my children's homes have been populated by a total of six Golden and five Labrador

Retrievers. Labs are, overwhelmingly, the most popular breed, not just in the UK but in the United States, Canada and elsewhere. I'm sure that's because they are the happiest dogs in all of dogdom and have brains the size of kumquats.

There were only a few loose ends to tie up at the clinic. Brenda quickly found a calm and equable blotched tabby cat for Dr Samuelson, not from Miss Wallace, as I'd expected, but through her jungle telegraph connections with other RANAs in London. Now that Keith and I weren't going to set up a joint practice with Richard, I had no specific plans but felt I shouldn't telephone people to tell them I was leaving, in case I ended up practising nearby. That would be akin to stealing clients from Bluey, but I did call John Gielgud and Martin Hensler, and Miss Wallace. Brian brought a bottle of wine to the surgery on my last day and we drank not just to my departure but to Pat's too. She had been with him since he first arrived and decided that working for anyone else would be second best. Pat and her husband were looking to become tenants in a pub in Devon.

I thought about returning to Ontario, but after three years in the heart of London, the idea of opening a clinic in a strip mall shopping centre in Toronto's suburbs wasn't appealing. And Julia's career was in London. That was a given. Could I, should I, uproot her from her career and move back to Canada? On the other hand, do you know how mind-numbingly miserable the weather is in London compared with southwestern Ontario?

I discussed with the two men who were my closest friends, David and Meredith, what I should do with my future. I also talked more with Keith.

David advised me to remain, as he had, in London.

'We're four hours by boat train from Paris or Amsterdam,' David commented. 'And the cost of living here is half what it is in Canada.'

Meredith tacked differently. 'You love the theatre. The theatre loves Julia. That seems to be a unique state of affairs. Will
you better it by returning to Canada?'

I decided it would be most fun setting up my own practice,
being my own boss.

Keith told me that a vet north of the Royal Parks might be
interested in selling his practice. That seemed perfect. London
is curiously parochial, and I knew that people living south of
the parks seldom ventured north of them and vice versa. It was
far enough away from Pont Street and also far from Keith,
Andrew or Michael Gordon in Bayswater. I went to visit the vet
who owned the surgery. He shocked me.

The surgery itself was in an impressive house just off Marble
Arch. The basement and ground floor had more space that Brian's
four floors. The first, second and third floors provided elegant
accommodation, certainly suitable for a family and a nanny.

I met the vet, a loud man with the gait of a farmer who was
routinely trodden on by his livestock, after he had finished his
morning appointments and before he started his operations. He
was a 'veterinary practitioner', someone who had not graduated
from a veterinary school but had learned his trade through
apprenticing with a vet. The Veterinary Surgeons Act of 1948
permitted these individuals to continue working as vets although
they had no formal qualifications.

He took me on a tour of his spacious facilities. In the kennel
room there was a whippet, admitted just before I arrived. The
vet had pinned a broken femur the previous week but either the
pin was too small or the dog had raced around like, well, a
whippet, and the pin was now protruding from the skin on the
dog's left hip.

'Fogle. Hold this dog tight to your chest.'

He put the dog in my arms and made a makeshift muzzle
with one-inch-wide gauze bandage. Whippets always have the

most plaintive look in their eyes, and this dog was no different. I was glad I was now holding it so close that I couldn't see those eyes.

'Hold it firmly. This will just take a second.'

The vet picked up a hammer and drove the pin back down under the skin. The dog shrieked with pain.

I couldn't believe what I'd seen, but in keeping with how I behaved at that time I said nothing and left as soon as I could. That evening when I picked up Julia from the theatre I told her what happened. She wanted me to drive straight to his surgery so that she could tell him directly what she thought of him, but calmed down when I said, 'I'm setting up practice as close as I can get to that bastard.'

That turned out to be a little more difficult than I thought, but not much. I visited the estate agents who handled the Hyde Park Estate for its owners, the Church of England.

'I'm terribly sorry but we can't offer you any of our available properties,' I am told. 'We already have a vet on the estate.'

'Yes, I know you do, but I'd like to offer local pet owners another choice,' I explain.

'That would be unfair to the resident vet,' the estate agent replies.

The other side of Edgware Road is owned by the Portman Estate. Even better, it had a superior postcode, W1. The Portman Estate had a property available with a fourteen-year lease on Seymour Street, a five-minute walk from the other vet's. Keith had told me it was best to own a property, not lease it, but 22 Seymour Street was absolutely magnificent, the end of an imposing Georgian terrace built in the late 1700s. It was a palace, and I set about finding the money to buy the lease. The fact that I could have bought three freehold homes in Fulham for the same price as a short lease in Marylebone didn't enter my mind. I had to have it.

There was the modest question of money. How could we afford to buy an expensive, five-floor, 3,000-square-foot, central London home? I had left my job and had no income, but Julia not only had excellent income for the last three years but the guarantee of further employment when *Notes on a Love Affair* finished its run. John and Lisel Gale, husband and wife theatrical producers, had already offered her a new play.

I went to my bank manager armed with Julia's accounts.

'You are a professional, so I will give you an 80 per cent mortgage on the short lease,' the bank manager tells me, 'but Julia is an actress, so I'm afraid I can't include her income in any decision I make. And she's still married to someone else, so technically the income is not hers. It's her husband's.'

In 1973 the Inland Revenue did not yet allow a married woman to file her own tax return. It had to be filed with her husband. Not only could we not use Julia's income to get a mortgage, I'd still have to find the money to convert the premises into a veterinary clinic, plus another £6,000 for the mortgage shortfall. And make sure Julia's divorce, on a back burner since I met her, got our full attention.

The first challenge was generously met when my friend David stepped in with the second mortgage, five years at zero per cent interest! The place would be ours. Working out how I'd kit out the surgery was something I'd think about later. The top priority now was Julia's divorce. She and her husband had been separated for over five years, so it was simply a paperwork challenge.

Her divorce came through on a Friday in early April, and with that out of the way I said, 'So, when should we get married?' Julia's response was just as unromantic.

'Well, I need to get in touch with Gina Fratini for a wedding dress. You've got those lectures in Cambridge you're going to on Tuesday and Wednesday, I've got matinees on Thursday and

Saturday, so how about Friday?' It was a Friday the thirteenth, but neither of us is superstitious. On Monday, I contacted the Kensington Registry Office, and Julia asked Marvin and Deborah if they would be our witnesses. Marvin told her he would organise some drinks for us afterwards.

On Friday 13 April 1973, with Emily our flower girl, Honey our ring bearer, and Marvin Liebman and Deborah Kerr our witnesses, Julia and I married at Kensington Registry Office. Julia was the darling of the press, so there were photos next day in all the tabloids and broadsheets of Julia beaming, Emily scowling and me with my full beard, as Frank Manolson had once told me, looking like an embarrassed Jesus.

Marvin's 'drinks' for us turned out to be a grand reception at the Carlton Towers hotel, two minutes from where I had worked on Pont Street. Julia, Emily, Honey and I walked through the foyer of the hotel, where I pointed out that Feliks Topolski, the artist who had produced the dramatic glass mural in the foyer, was the same Feliks Topolski who sketched my caricature two years previously in a charity fund-raising event in Belgrave Square Gardens. 'Then if it's valuable you should have it framed and sell it to raise money for your surgery,' Julia sensibly replied.

We entered the Garden Room to vigorous applause. The guests sure knew what actors revered. The entire company from *Notes on a Love Affair*, stage crew, actors, office staff from Marvin's Sedgemoor Productions and his friends from other productions were there. We worked our way through the crowd. Marvin introduced us once more to Miss Nancy McLarty from Vero Beach, one of his investors. Nancy enjoyed the gathering so much that in future years she organised an annual dinner for all her theatrical friends in London.

He introduced us to Ingrid Bergman.

'Ingrid is really Jewish,' he told us. 'That's why she's so beautiful. Her mother Friedel Adler was German, like my mother.'

'I hope you don't mind that I gatecrashed,' Miss Bergman explained. 'Deborah told me she was going to be a witness at your wedding, and I love weddings, so I asked her if she thought you would mind if I came.'

Julia introduced me to Coral Browne, an elegant Australian actress, my mother's age, whom she had worked with previously. In turn, Coral introduced us to the American actor Vincent Price.

'Are you working together?' I asked.

'He's my fucking lover,' Coral coolly replied. Vincent, holding her small Yorkie in his arms, added, 'We're working together in a film, *Theatre with Blood*. I love it. It's the closest I'll ever be allowed to get to true Shakespearean acting.'

Julia and I chatted with the guests, alternately keeping Honey, unused to being on a lead, with one of us. After an hour I thought it best to take her outside for a pee break and met Vincent, doing the same with Coral's Yorkie.

'Bruce, you are a vet. Would you like this fucking dog?' was his greeting. We had both been given keys to Cadogan Place Gardens and took our dogs in, where I let Honey off her lead. Vincent kept Coral's on a short tether. 'If anything happens to this fucking dog, it's the end of a beautiful friendship. Have you known Marvin for a long time?'

I explained I'd only met him six months previously but that he was a generous and warm-hearted man.

'He is the beating heart of the conservative movement in America,' Vincent told me. 'William F. Buckley's godson. Knows absolutely everyone. A convert to Catholicism. It's such a surprise to discover he's producing films and plays.'

I was amazed. I thought Marvin was a typical New York Jewish liberal.

'So exactly what did he do before what he's doing now?' I asked, and Vincent told me Marvin was the most successful fundraiser for anti-communist and conservative movements in the world.

'He is a fierce anti-communist. He was secretary of the Committee of One Million Against the Admission of Red China to the United Nations. He gave up two years ago when they finally got admitted.'

'So why do you think he's here?' I asked.

'All his friends are brutally conservative anti-communists. What's wonderful is they all know Marvin is as queer as a pink possum but they all still love him and give him their money, even for his West End plays it seems.'

'I haven't seen any sign of a boyfriend,' I said, and Vincent replied, 'There won't be one until he's honest with himself – and becomes a Jew again.'

Twenty years later, Marvin did just that, and wrote an auto-biography called *Coming Out Conservative*.

'Shall we go back in?' Vincent suggested. 'I'd like to meet your parents.'

Two days before, Julia's father Dick had experienced a mild heart attack. His doctor told him not to attend the wedding, and his wife Jean and mother-in-law Matt decided that if one couldn't go, none would. I didn't have such a noble excuse with my own parents.

'Actually, none of our parents are here, but you've reminded me to call mine.' And with Julia, Emily and Honey by my side, from a pay phone in the lobby of the Carlton Towers hotel I phoned my mother to tell her we just got married.

Looking back now at my relationship with my parents, at my thinking that my dad was an empty vessel and only learning through his letters that he just worked differently to me, and at my mother, how we wounded each other in the most pointless ways, all of that with time disappears like a morning mist.

I must say Mum was charming on the telephone and was hurt, not because we married but because we did so without giving her the opportunity to attend. I felt like a heel and told her we would honeymoon in New York once Julia's play finished, then come to Toronto and have another marriage ceremony for the family there.

Julia's play was in fact running out of steam and Marvin closed it down the following month. In late May, Julia and I flew to New York, staying in John Gielgud's apartment overlooking Central Park. He not only gave us his apartment for our honeymoon, he provided us with a housekeeper who each day filled, and I mean totally filled, the apartment with fresh flowers. I felt as if we were living in my father's flower shop. Julia the romantic loved the theatricality of John's warmhearted and welcoming gesture.

After a week in New York we flew to Toronto, where my mother had organised a wedding ceremony, with herself and my Uncle Reub as our witnesses, then a family reception in her home. Just as she had orchestrated two of her brothers to write and advise me not to marry Julia, now she had instructed them to accept Julia into her family. Our second marriage in two months was as wonderful as our first.

Soon after we got back from New York and Toronto, Julia visited John and Lisel Gale to find out more about the play they had offered her. The Gale's great commercial success, *No Sex Please, We're British*, had been playing to consistently full houses for the last three years at the Strand Theatre. Julia returned from her meeting with them bubbling with excitement.

'It was called *Avanti* on Broadway but John is going to call it *A Touch of Spring* here,' she explains to me over dinner.

'A good role?' I ask.

'Well, Sandy and Diana are in Rome to collect Sandy's father's corpse. Diana is very irritating and has wonderfully funny lines like, "Can't anyone turn off those church bells?" and huffs back to America. Alison – that's me – is English and also in Rome to pick up her mother's corpse. She was killed in the same car accident and Sandy is the only one who immediately works out they were lovers. I'm fresh and funny and enchanting, and I charm Sandy out of his stodgy rut. Yes, it's a wonderful role, and there's a local fixer, Baldo, who lusts after both Sandy and me, so it's great fun. Very commedia dell'arte.'

'Written by anyone I've heard of?' I ask.

'I had to admit to John and Lisel that I'd never heard of Samuel Taylor, but he wrote the screenplays for *Vertigo* with James Stewart and *Sabrina* with Audrey Hepburn. And his real name is Samuel Tannenbaum, so he's probably one more of your distant relatives. I've agreed to do it and we start rehearsals in a month.'

In late June we completed the formalities of acquiring the lease to Seymour Street and moved into the roomy upstairs three-floor flat – four bedrooms, a double lounge and a spacious kitchen. We now had room to invite people to *our* home for dinner and did so with gusto. Our first guests were John Gielgud and Martin Hensler. They brought their three dogs with them. John was in the midst of a flurry of theatrical productions. He had a revival of Noël Coward's *Private Lives* running, starring Maggie Smith and her husband John Stephens, and was about to direct Ingrid Bergman in W. Somerset Maugham's *Constant Wife* at the Albery Theatre.

'Incredible casting. No man vould have affair if he married to Ingrid,' Martin says.

'I hear she speaks five languages and can't act in any of them,' John replies, then adds, 'But that doesn't matter. Audiences adore her. Martin adores her. I adore her.'

'Ve bomped into Margaret, the sexy Duchess,' Martin added. 'Ve tell her when you open for business.'

Frank and Jackie Marcus lived a short walk away and became regular guests, but we were especially pleased that Diana and Moragh Bernard accepted an invitation to dinner and brought Anna their Pug, whom our dog Honey found very amusing to paw and play with. We told them we were planning to fit in a long weekend in Venice before *A Touch of Spring* opened and they gave us a list of things we must do, where to stay, out-of-the-way churches to visit, places to be at a certain time of day to capture a fleeting reflection of light, not just where to eat but what to ask for that wasn't on the menu. Julia was prepared to give them anything of ours that they told us they liked but they only commented on Honey, and that would have been a step much too far for Julia.

Finding equipment for my new business was much easier than getting planning permission to change the use of the basement, ground and first floor from dental to veterinary surgery. The City of Westminster told me they were short-staffed and could not review my application for eighteen months. I mentioned that to Sir John, he told me he would look into it, and two weeks later my application was approved. I don't know what he did. There was a similar problem with the Post Office. They told me they could not instal a new telephone system until late 1974, over a year later. Again, I mentioned that to John, and by September we got the two lines we needed, a private one upstairs and a business one with three extensions downstairs, with a further extension by our bed for use when I was on emergency call.

Growing up in Canada, I found the British use of the word 'surgery' for a medical, dental or veterinary office, or a politician's office for that matter, odd, even uncomfortable. I preferred the North American 'clinic'. Surgeries were invariably given the names of the vets working in them, if only because the Royal College of Veterinary Surgeons prohibited us from using either street or district names. I couldn't call my new practice the

Seymour Street Veterinary Clinic or the Marylebone Veterinary
Clinic but thought I might get away with naming it after my
landlord, and registered it as the Portman Veterinary Clinic.

Julia contacted Dulux, and they provided paint and wallpaper of our choosing (well, Julia's choosing) for the fifteen
rooms of the house, as well as the unending hallways and stucco
exterior. In return, they wanted pictures of Julia decorating her
house with their products.

Because it had been a dental surgery for seventy years, there
were taps and sinks everywhere I needed them, in the basement
and in both rooms on the first floor. I didn't have to undertake
any plumbing or electrical wiring, just the decorating, then
equipping.

I sold the Rembrandt etching I bought at Harrods (but not the
Renoir or the Topolski), and with that money travelled to
Yorkshire, where a vet had a barn filled with American Armed
Forces surplus medical equipment from the Vietnam War, which
was then starting to wind down. The surgical instruments were the
world's finest. Some lasted over forty years. The vet had a portable
electrocardiograph in a camouflage box. I bought that too.

When I returned from Yorkshire, Julia suggested that we go
around the corner to Biaggi's, the local Italian restaurant Frank
and Jackie had introduced us to. I knew from her dancing eyes
she wanted to tell me something.

'Let's have champagne,' she suggests. With our glasses filled,
she looks at me, reaches out, holds my hand and says, 'I'm
pregnant!'

'Wow,' I answer. 'A little bit pregnant or a whole lot
pregnant?'

'My ankles are weak. They keep bending over,' she replies.
'That's what happened when I was pregnant with Emily. And I
haven't had a migraine for almost two months.'

'I thought your doctor said the copper coil would prevent pregnancies.'

'Well, I guess the baby will have a toy to play with,' Julia replies.

'So that means you can help decorate the house?' I query. 'What will you tell John Gale?'

'What will *we* tell John Gale,' Julia responds. 'You're coming with me.'

The next morning Julia telephones John Gale and we go to see him that afternoon. Lisel his wife and co-producer is petite, short-haired and quiet. John is a wonderful counterpoint to her, a big, loud, ebullient man. He gives both of us bear hugs as we enter his office.

'Have some champagne, darlings,' he says, and pours each of us a glass.

'To *A Touch of Magic*,' he toasts, giving the play a mild name change.

After some small talk he says, 'Now, darlings. What do you want to see me about?' To which Julia replies, 'Bruce has something he wants to tell you.' They turn to me and I say, 'John, Lisel, I'm happy to say that Julia's pregnant but sad to say that because she is she won't be able to fulfil her contract with you.'

'Isn't that wonderful!' Lisel responds, but John is silent.

He gets up from his chair and comes over to me. I'm tall but John is taller, and has girth.

'Bruce, stand up,' he commands, and I do.

He grabs me by both shoulders and unblinkingly stares straight into my eyes.

'Bruce, you've fucked us both!'

He kisses me, on the lips. 'Congratulations!' he roars. 'Have more champagne!'

POSTSCRIPT

John Gale produced *A Touch of Spring* the following year, with Hayley Mills taking the part Julia had to forfeit. Julian Fellowes and Leigh Lawson co-starred. Hayley and Leigh had a son soon after, around the same time Julia and I had our daughter, Tamara.

Dulux came to take photos of Julia decorating our home, but because she was by then visibly pregnant they didn't use them.

When the lease on Brian's premises expired, it ceased being a veterinary surgery and became a women's fashion shop. Brian was later appointed a CBE for services to the veterinary profession.

Pat and her husband became successful publicans.

Frank Manolson died of heart and liver disease five years later, only fifty-three years old, and is buried in Oxford.

Christopher closed down Town & Country Dogs. He continues to source pups for his old clients and boards them in his home in Wiltshire.

Harrods stopped selling wildlife soon after I left Brian's but continued selling dogs and cats for another forty years until the pet department permanently closed in 2014.

Annabelle joined me as my first nurse at the Portman Veterinary Clinic.

Our son Ben was born at the end of 1973.

Keith Butt, Andrew Carmichael, Michael Gordon and I formed a business partnership. Keith died in 2019 and the rest of us are still in practice. We have had cumulatively over 230 years of clinical experience. My surviving partners still treat me like the baby.

ACKNOWLEDGEMENTS

Time can play tricks on your mind, and remembering back fifty years is bound to be imaginative as well as factual. I'm grateful for the help of many who have ensured that at least some of the fact is accurate, especially Christopher Grievson and my veterinary partners Keith Butt, Michael Gordon and Andrew Carmichael. Other vets, including Peter Bedford, Gary Clayton Jones and Bruce Jones, the latter two from the Veterinary History Society (and Bruce a contemporary of Brian Singleton), also helped with fact checking.

I continue to learn about dog, cat and people behaviour from the nurses, vets, clients and clients' pets I meet at work. Thanks to all of you. Curiously, it's been fascinating seeing pets in their own homes, now that I'm unexpectedly meeting so many online rather than at the clinic. It's added another level of understanding, seeing exactly how our buddies behave on their own territory.

Special thanks to Hannah Macdonald, formerly of HarperCollins. Hannah was the first person to read the initial draft of this book, and she gave me her usual intelligent and lucid observations.

Thanks, too, to the English weather, always a great inducement to stay inside and write, and also to my family, especially my wife Julia, who has always encouraged me, from my first longhand manuscript forty years ago, through many 'how to' books about dogs and cats, to this reminiscence.